T0304591

Grant writing for medical and healthcare professionals

Subhash Chandra Parija • Vikram Kate
Editors

Grant writing for medical and healthcare professionals

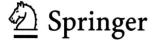 Springer

Editors
Subhash Chandra Parija
Sri Balaji Vidyapeeth University
Pondicherry, India

Vikram Kate
Department of General and Gastrointestinal surgery
Jawaharlal Institute of Postgraduate Medical Education and Research (JIPMER)
Pondicherry, India

ISBN 978-981-19-7020-7   ISBN 978-981-19-7018-4   (eBook)
https://doi.org/10.1007/978-981-19-7018-4

This Springer imprint is published by the registered company Springer Nature Singapore Pte Ltd.
The registered company address is: 152 Beach Road, #21-01/04 Gateway East, Singapore 189721, Singapore

Dedicated to ....
My Father Late Shri. Managovinda Parija
Mother Late Smt. Nishamani Parija
Wife Ms. Jyotirmayee Parija
and
my Professional Colleagues and Mentors
Subhash Chandra Parija

My family
Nina,
Anahita, Niroj, little Nyra
Anuraag, Haritha,
and
to my dear students, colleagues, and above all
my mentors
Vikram Kate

Foreword

I am extremely delighted to write this Foreword for the book entitled *Grant Writing for Medical and Healthcare Professionals* being compiled and edited by Prof. S C Parija and Prof. Vikram Kate. From conception of an idea, to plan a research study, to generate essential resources and then implement the plan(s) are all essential ingredients in any type of research including medical, biomedical, and public health aspects. All will agree that this path of research is fraught with difficulties. These problems stem from both logistical issues and from scientific hitches of the task at hand. Solving them requires sound domain knowledge, expertise of the field, choosing right strategies, the presence of a support team of competent collaborators, assistants, and monetary backing. These components are crucial to ensure the smooth sailing of any project, however, securing them often poses a challenge. Although institutional support can sometimes suffice, its access is not universal. This is where a research grant comes into play. It allows the researcher to obtain the required resources, which in turn renders him/her independent. This permits the researcher(s) to expand their thought process and foray into unknown areas without being tethered by bureaucratic or fiscal restrictions.

Despite the obvious benefits of grant writing and getting assured funding support, very few venture into this world and an even smaller number succeed in it. This is primarily because they find the task of writing a grant daunting, hazy, and very little is available out there that details the basics and the nuances. This book entitled *Grant Writing for Medical and Healthcare Professionals* by Prof. Parija and Prof. Kate aims to demystify this herculean task and does a superlative job at that. Their book has a very systematic approach and has examined the task of grant writing from every facet—the prospective writer, the funding organizations, and the different intricacies involved. This book has highly informative and stimulating 21 chapters on diverse yet important aspects of grant writing. Not only basic fundamental aspects useful to compete for grants from Indian agencies are well covered, but this book also gives important information to those who wish to compete for research grants in the USA, UK, Australia, and important Asian countries.

Prof. Parija and Prof. Kate are renowned experts in their respective fields and on the current subject matter. Prof. Parija is a recipient of the B C Roy National Award of the Medical Council of India for his contribution to the development of Medical Microbiology. Prof. Kate, a recipient of the "Distinguished DNB Teacher of

Excellence Award" of the Association of National Board Accredited Institutions has contributed a large number of chapters in reputed textbooks of surgical gastroenterology and surgery in national and international textbooks along with numerous papers to his credit. The joint venture of these two doyens has resulted in successful works on *Writing and Publishing a Scientific Research Paper* and *Thesis Writing for Master's and PhD Program*. These texts have helped several enthusiastic young researchers voyage into the world of academia. This textbook follows the same trend and shall no doubt be the third of an impressive hat-trick! I hope that this book will help the hesitant researchers to shed the reluctance that prevents them from grant writing! I am sure the book will be found useful both by emerging young and established serious researchers and can be referred to every time they encounter a rough patch or they wish to empower themselves with better ideas and useful tips. I compliment the authors as well as editors for this excellent effort. I am highly optimistic that we will see many editions of this book in the coming years to fulfill the emerging needs of researchers in health sciences.

JIPMER   V. M. Katoch
Pondicherry, India

AIIMS
Madurai, Tamil Nadu, India

Lepra Society
Essex, UK

Department of Health Research, Government of India
New Delhi, India

Indian Council of Medical Research
New Delhi, India

Public Health Research, Rajasthan University of Health
Sciences (RUHS)
Jaipur, Rajasthan, India

Preface

The path traversed by any student typically begins with primary school which then progresses through secondary school and finally culminates into college. In the medical field, this is usually followed by a postgraduate degree course after which most individuals then embark into the world of their professional development. A few wish to further specialize and these individuals are those with carefully chosen niche areas which they want to delve further into and master. A similar analogy can be derived from this and applied to the world of research wherein a novice person would start out with understanding research methodology and the nuances of writing a paper. With growing experience, they would start to publish their own research and mentor people keen on venturing into academic publishing. It is a select group of individuals, not unlike the cohort who wish to super-specialize, who take that extra step forward and attempt grant-writing. This book entitled *Grant Writing for Medical and Healthcare Professionals* aims to demystify this herculean task and does a superlative job at that.

The content of this book is organized into sections that eases the flow of understanding and provides a concise overview of the individuals topics. The book is carefully prepared keeping in mind the difficulties faced by the young researchers. The details on choosing a funding agency, grant makers' expectations, budgeting, surveillance and site visits, rights of the researchers, ethical and legal aspects of obtaining the grant have been covered extensively. The book also includes on how to report the source of funding, acknowledgment, good clinical practice guidelines, and the nuances on dealing with the rejected grant proposal.

With a total of 21 chapters, each component of grant writing has been included, which not only covers basics such as the purpose of grant writing and understanding the funding agencies but also the expected follow-up and Good Clinical Practice Guidelines. By adding a separate discussion on dealing with rejected grant proposals, we have addressed perhaps the most common reason as to why young researchers quit grant writing. This special perspective provides an added dimension into the real-life struggle of dealing with grant writing. Furthermore, the book is inclusive in its approach to grant writing by focusing not only on the national but also international agencies of funding. A handy checklist has also been incorporated within the contents and can act as a ready reckoner before the final submissions to ensure that the grant proposal is not hindered by technical insufficiencies.

Pondicherry, India   Subhash Chandra Parija
                                                                                      Vikram Kate

Acknowledgments

First of all, our thanks go to the participants and the authors of this book. We would like to thank all the authors for their contribution to the scientific content and preparation of this book. We would like to express our deep gratitude to Dr. Vigneshvar Chandrasekaran, Assistant Professor, Department of Psychiatry, Mahatma Gandhi Medical College and Research Institute, Sri Balaji Vidyapeeth, Puducherry for his exceedingly committed editorial assistance throughout the preparation of this book. These include receiving the manuscripts, assembling the contents and its review, and coordination with the authors. Our appreciation and gratitude to Dr. Kalayarasan, Additional Professor and Head, Department of Surgical Gastroenterology, Dr. Suresh Kumar, Professor of Surgery, both at the Jawaharlal Institute of Postgraduate Medical Education and Research (JIPMER), Puducherry, for their editorial assistance and a methodical review of this project right from the stage of inception.

We are grateful to Dr. Anahita Kate, Faculty-Cornea and Anterior Segment Services, L V Prasad Eye Institute, Vijayawada, Dr. Gurushankari Balakrishnan, Senior Resident, Department of Surgery, JIPMER, Puducherry, India and Dr. Sejal Jain, Junior Resident, Department of Dermatology, Venereology and Leprology, Postgraduate Institute of Medical Education and Research (PGIMER), Chandigarh for the editorial assistance, assembling the text, proof reading, and making this into a coherent manuscript.

We are grateful to Ms. Srijita Saha, Ms. Aarushi Kollana, and Ms. Himadri Sarkar, MBBS students, JIPMER, Puducherry, for providing wonderful cartoons for the chapters, which made the book look more reader friendly. Last but not least, we would like to thank the publisher, Springer Nature, for the association and for helping to bring out this book for the readers.

Subhash Chandra Parija

Vikram Kate

Contents

Editors and Contributors

About the Editors

Subhash Chandra Parija MBBS, MD, PhD, DSc, FRCPath is currently the Vice-Chancellor of Shri Balaji Vidyapeeth, Pondicherry. He was the former Director and also Dean (Research) of the Jawaharlal Institute of Postgraduate Medical Education and Research (JIPMER), Pondicherry. He obtained MBBS (1977) from Utkal University, Cuttack; MD (Microbiology) (1981) from Banaras Hindu University (BHU), Varanasi; PhD (Microbiology) (1987) from the University of Madras, Chennai. He is one of the very few Medical Microbiologists of India to be conferred DSc (Microbiology), highest degree in research, for his contribution in the field of Medical Parasitology by the University of Madras, Chennai. Prof. Parija was conferred with the Distinguished BHU Alumnus Award in the field of Medical Sciences.

Prof. Parija has nearly four decades of teaching and research experience, contributing mainly to infectious diseases, especially parasitology, diagnostics, and public health. He is actively involved in conducting research programs on immunology, epidemiology, and simple, cost-effective diagnostic tests for parasitic diseases in the community and low resource settings.

Prof. Parija, author of more than 400 research papers, has supervised more than 85 PhD, MD, and other postgraduate theses as supervisor and co-supervisor; has 23 copy rights, 1 patent granted and another 1 patent published; and transferred one technology in commercialization of a product. He has authored/edited 16 books including most popular *Textbook of Medical Parasitology*, and the most recent *Effective Medical Communication, The A,B,C,D,E of it* published by Springer.

Prof. Parija is a Fellow of the Royal College of Pathologists, London; and International Academy of Medical Sciences, New Delhi. He is also a Fellow of many professional bodies of eminence such as the National Academy of Medical Sciences, New Delhi; the Indian College of Pathologists, New Delhi; the Indian Academy of Tropical Parasitology, Pondicherry and many others. In recognition of his immense contributions in research in parasitic diseases, Prof. Parija has been honored with more than 26 awards both international and national such as Dr. B C Roy National Award of the Medical Council of India, BPKIHS Internal Oration Award, Dr R V Rajam Oration Award of the National Academy of Medical

Sciences, Distinguished BHU Alumni Award of the Banaras Hindu University, Dr. S C Agarwal Oration Award of the Indian Association of Medical Microbiologists, Dr. B P Pandey Memorial Oration Award of the Indian Association of Medical Microbiologists, etc.

Among others, Prof. Parija founded the Indian Academy of Tropical Parasitology, launched a Scientific Journal *Tropical Parasitology*, initiated a quality assurance program in diagnostic parasitology, also founded Health and Intellectual Property Rights Academy to promote Intellectual Property Rights activities in Health Sciences; and mentored students both undergraduates, postgraduates, PhD scholars, and young faculty to pursue their interest and career in parasitic diseases of public health importance.

The current areas of his interest include e-governance, integration of communication technology in medical health care, and medical education including effective medical communication.

Vikram Kate MS, FRCS (Eng.), FRCS (Ed.), FRCS (Glasg), Ph.D., is presently working as a Senior Professor of General and Gastrointestinal Surgery at the Jawaharlal Institute of Postgraduate Medical Education and Research (JIPMER) Pondicherry, India. Prof. Kate was awarded PhD in Surgical Gastroenterology for his pioneering doctoral work on *Helicobacter pylori* and its correlation with perforated duodenal ulcer. He has contributed to more than 45 chapters in reputed textbooks of surgical gastroenterology and surgery and has more than 200 papers to his credit.

He is bestowed with the prestigious honor of being the Inaugural President of the Indian Chapter of *Society for the Surgery of the Alimentary Tract* (SSAT), USA (2021–2022) and the Member of the Research Committee of the *Society for Surgery of the Alimentary Tract (SSAT),* USA (2020–2023). He is also a Member of the *Surgical Specialty Board-General Surgery* of The Royal College of Surgeons of Edinburgh, UK (2021–2024) and the Past President of the *Indian Association of Surgical Gastroenterology.* In recognition of his work, Prof. Kate was awarded the prestigious *Distinguished DNB Teacher of Excellence Award* for the year 2018 of the Association of National Board Accredited Institutions and the *Great Contributor Award* for the year 2021 for excellence and contribution to the field of Research and Conference Presentations by the Association of Minimal Access Surgeons of India (AMASI).

He is the recipient of many prestigious oration awards such as *Dr. Mathias Oration–2010* and the *Prof. N. Rangabashyam Oration–2015* instituted by the Tamil Nadu and Pondicherry Chapter of the Association of Surgeons of India, the *Veerabai JR Das Oration–2016* by the Indian Association of Surgical Gastroenterology, the Dr. *S K Bhansali Memorial Oration–2017* by the Association of Surgeons of India, *Annual Internal Oration–2015* of the JIPMER Scientific Society and the *Senior Faculty Research Oration–2020* of JIPMER, First *Dr. Indru Khubchandani Oration–2020* by the International Society of Colo-Proctology and the *Puducherry ASI Oration Award–2021* of the Puducherry Chapter of Association of Surgeons of India. He has also won more than 75 best paper awards for his papers and work at the international and national conferences including the prestigious *Residents and Fellows Research Conference Presentation Award for 2021 by the* Society *for Surgery of the Alimentary Tract*, USA. Prof. Kate is associated with various committees in the capacity as Examiner for the Intercollegiate Board of Surgery of the Royal College of Surgeons, Edinburgh and England and is associated with the MS/DNB program in surgery and MCh program for GI Surgery. He is also an Inspector for GI Surgery for the National Board of Examinations.

Prof. Kate is the Editor-in-Chief of the journal *International Journal of Advanced Medical and Health Research*, an official publication of JIPMER, Puducherry and *Chief Editor for Medscape Reference Gastrointestinal Procedures Section* of the prestigious medical website of *Medscape Reference* of WebMD, Omaha USA and has also contributed many articles to *Medscape Reference*. Prof. Kate in collaboration with Prof. Parija edited books on *Writing and Publishing a Scientific Paper and Thesis Writing for Master's and PhD Program*, which was published by Springer Nature in 2017 and 2018, respectively. He has contributed chapters to *Textbooks of Surgical Gastroenterology* (Edited by S. Haribhakti; PK Mishra) *Gastrointestinal Surgery Annual* Published by the Indian Association of Surgical Gastroenterology, *Roshan Lall Gupta's Recent Advances in Surgery* and *Bailey & Love's Essential Operations in Hepatobiliary and Pancreatic Surgery*.

Prof. Kate is also on the Editorial Board of some international and national journals such as *Gastroenterology Research and Practice* and *Indian Journal of Surgery*. He successfully published a Special Issue on *Helicobacter pylori infection and Upper Gastrointestinal Disorders* as a Lead Editor for *Gastroenterology Research and Practice* and is a Peer Reviewer for many National and International Journals including the Cochrane Review. He is a Fellow of Royal college of Surgeons of England (FRCS), Edinburgh (FRCSEd.), and Glasgow (FRCSGlasg.) and the Faculty of Surgical Trainers of Edinburgh (FFSTEd.). He is in receipt of the prestigious American Fellowships and is a Fellow of the American College of Surgeons (FACS), Fellow of the American College of Gastroenterology (FACG), and a Member of the American Society of Colon and Rectal Surgeons (MASCRS).

Contributors

Khaled Altarrah Faculty of Medicine, University of Birmingham, Birmingham, UK
Ibn Sina Specialist Hospital, Ministry of Health, Kuwait City, Kuwait

Gurushankari Balakrishnan Department of Surgery, Jawaharlal Institute of Postgraduate Medical Education and Research (JIPMER), Pondicherry, India

Savio George Barreto Hepatopancreatobiliary and Liver Transplant Unit, Division of Surgery and Perioperative Medicine, Flinders Medical Centre, Adelaide, SA, Australia

Vigneshvar Chandrasekaran Department of Psychiatry, Mahatma Gandhi Medical College and Research Institute, Sri Balaji Vidyapeeth, Pondicherry, India

Biswajit Dubashi Department of Medical Oncology, Jawaharlal Institute of Postgraduate Medical Education and Research (JIPMER), Pondicherry, India

Prasanth Ganesan Department of Medical Oncology, Jawaharlal Institute of Postgraduate Medical Education and Research (JIPMER), Pondicherry, India

Rajesh Nachiappa Ganesh Department of Pathology, Jawaharlal Institute of Post-Graduate Medical Education and Research (JIPMER), Pondicherry, India

Nirmal Kumar Ganguly Indian Council of Medical Research, New Delhi, India
Apollo Hospitals Educational and Research Foundation (AHERF), New Delhi, India

Luxitaa Goenka Department of Medical Oncology, Jawaharlal Institute of Postgraduate Medical Education and Research (JIPMER), Pondicherry, India

Divya Gupta Department of Dermatology, Dr. B.R. Ambedkar Medical College, Bengaluru, India
Division of Pediatric Dermatology, Manipal Hospitals, Bengaluru, India

Wei Hong Lai Clinical Research Centre, Institute for Clinical Research, Sarawak General Hospital, Jalan Hospital, Kuching, Sarawak, Malaysia

Rajive Mathew Jose Plastic and Hand Surgery, University Hospital Birmingham, Birmingham, UK

Mitwa Joshi Faculty of Medicine, Nursing and Health Sciences, Monash University, Clayton, VIC, Australia

Prashant Joshi Department of Surgery, School of Clinical Sciences at Monash Health, Monash University, Clayton, VIC, Australia
Department of Cardiothoracic Surgery, Monash Health, Clayton, VIC, Australia

Shubhum Joshi Department of Neurosurgery, St Vincent's Hospital, Fitzroy, VIC, Australia

R. Kalayarasan Department of Surgical Gastroenterology, Jawaharlal Institute of Post-Graduate Medical Education and Research (JIPMER), Pondicherry, India

Vikram Kate Department of General and Gastrointestinal surgery, Jawaharlal Institute of Postgraduate Medical Education and Research (JIPMER), Pondicherry, India

Upninder Kaur Department of Medical Parasitology, Postgraduate Institute of Medical Education and Research (PGIMER), Chandigarh, India

Vaishali Londhe Department of Anaesthesia, Royal Victorian Eye and Ear Hospital, Melbourne, VIC, Australia

Avin Muthuramalingam Department of Psychiatry, Jawaharlal Institute of Postgraduate Medical Education and Research (JIPMER), Karaikal, India

Subhash Chandra Parija Sri Balaji Vidyapeeth, Pondicherry, India

Tae-kyung Park Medical Education, University Hospital Birmingham, Birmingham, UK

Satish G. Patil SDM College of Medical Sciences and Hospital, Shri Dharmasthala Manjunatheshwara University, Dharwad, Karnataka, India

Manju Rahi Division of Epidemiology and Communicable Diseases, Indian Council of Medical Research, New Delhi, India

Medha Rajappa Department of Biochemistry, Jawaharlal Institute of Postgraduate Medical Education and Research (JIPMER), Pondicherry, India

Balamurugan Ramadass Clinical Biochemistry Laboratory, Department of Biochemistry, Center of Excellence for Clinical Microbiome Research, All India Institute of Medical Sciences (AIIMS) Bhubaneswar, Bhubaneswar, Odisha, India

Gautam Kumar Saha Apollo Hospitals Educational and Research Foundation (AHERF), New Delhi, India

Asri bin Said Sarawak Heart Centre, Kuching-Samarahan Expressway, Kota Samarahan, Sarawak, Malaysia
Faculty of Medicine and Health Sciences, University Malaysia Sarawak, Jalan Datuk Mohammad Musa, Kota Samarahan, Sarawak, Malaysia

David J. Schneider Cardiovascular Research Institute, University of Vermont, Burlington, VT, USA

Rakesh Sehgal Department of Medical Parasitology, Postgraduate Institute of Medical Education and Research (PGIMER), Chandigarh, India

Devyani Sharma Department of Medical Parasitology, Postgraduate Institute of Medical Education and Research (PGIMER), Chandigarh, India

Sachin Sharma Indian Council of Medical Research, New Delhi, India

Toishi Sharma University of Vermont, Burlington, VT, USA

Shree Lakshmi Devi Singaravelu Shri Sathya Sai Medical College and Research Institute, Sri Balaji Vidyapeeth, Chengalpet, Tamil Nadu, India

Saurabh RamBihariLal Shrivastava Department of Community Medicine, Shri Sathya Sai Medical College and Research Institute, Sri Balaji Vidyapeeth, Chengalpet, Tamil Nadu, India

Julian A. Smith Department of Surgery, School of Clinical Sciences at Monash Health, Monash University, Clayton, VIC, Australia
Department of Cardiothoracic Surgery, Monash Health, Clayton, VIC, Australia

A. R. Srinivasan Biochemistry Department, Mahatma Gandhi Medical College and Research Institute, Sri Balaji Vidyapeeth, Pondicherry, India

Karthick Subramanian Department of Psychiatry, Mahatma Gandhi Medical College and Research Institute, Sri Balaji Vidyapeeth, Pondicherry, India

Sathasivam Sureshkumar Department of Surgery, Jawaharlal Institute of Post-Graduate Medical Education and Research (JIPMER), Pondicherry, India

Bhawna Yadav Indian Council of Medical Research, New Delhi, India

Alan Yean Yip Fong Clinical Research Centre, Institute for Clinical Research, Sarawak General Hospital, Jalan Hospital, Kuching, Sarawak, Malaysia
Sarawak Heart Centre, Kuching-Samarahan Expressway, Kota Samarahan, Sarawak, Malaysia

Part I

Understanding Grant Writing

What Is Your Aim (Ambition-Interest-Mission), and What You Want to Do?

1

Subhash Chandra Parija and Saurabh RamBihariLal Shrivastava

> *Without dreams and goals, there is no living, only merely existing, and that is not why we are here*
>
> *Mark Twain*

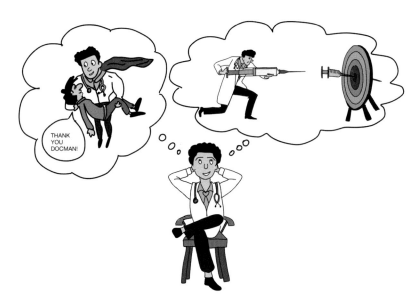

What is your AIM and what you want to achieve in health care

S. C. Parija (✉)
Sri Balaji Vidyapeeth, Pondicherry, India

S. R. Shrivastava
Department of Community Medicine, Shri Sathya Sai Medical College and Research Institute, Sri Balaji Vidyapeeth, Chengalpet, Tamil Nadu, India

© The Author(s), under exclusive license to Springer Nature Singapore Pte Ltd. 2023
S. C. Parija, V. Kate (eds.), *Grant writing for medical and healthcare professionals*,
https://doi.org/10.1007/978-981-19-7018-4_1

Objectives
- Understand the various roles of a medical teacher.
- Comprehend the role of research in enhancing academics and improving patient care.
- Realize the need for funding and grants in research.

1.1   Introduction

The field of medicine and delivery of medical education is quite complex, wherein the healthcare professionals are expected to perform a wide range of activities while discharging their duties [1]. The medical teachers have to become the change agent amid the paradigm shift being reported in the medical education delivery system [1]. The presence of a well-trained medical teacher is the essence of accomplishing our aim to ensure the successful implementation of curricular reforms and their sustainment [1, 2]. The medical teachers should be looked upon as not only someone who is an information provider but also someone who ensures comprehensive development of the students and, at the same time, makes significant gains on the professional front [1, 2].

1.2   Roles of a Medical Teacher

A medical teacher is expected to perform a wide range of activities about their specialty [2]. However, in the broad sense, these responsibilities can be categorized into Academics, Patient Care, and Research [2, 3]. The administration domain can also be considered one of the responsibilities. It is essential that as the medical teacher gains teaching experience, they simultaneously also should demonstrate their outcome in some or the other forms of administration (Fig. 1.1) [4]. The weightage of these roles can vary between different types of departments (viz., patient care

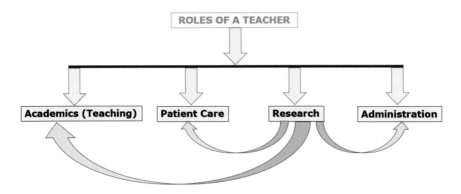

Fig. 1.1 Roles of a teacher

becomes an essential component for clinical departments, but the same benchmark cannot be drawn for preclinical departments) [3, 4].

1.2.1   Medical Teacher: Academics

In the real sense, transforming a recently joined student in a medical college into a competent medical graduate requires immense effort [5]. This is predominantly because we are not only looking to produce a graduate who possesses the desired knowledge and skills but should also develop critical thinking, clinical reasoning, and problem-solving skills [5, 6]. In addition, the students should acquire the traits of being professional, a leader, a team member, a good communicator, self-directed, and lifelong learners [7]. All these traits are pretty complex, and they will essentially require consistent and dedicated efforts from the teachers' side [7].

In academics, the first and foremost role of medical teachers is that they have to be information providers in both large group settings and small group settings. This even applies to teaching in practical or clinical settings [5, 7]. The teacher has to be a facilitator of learning through mentoring and guiding students to improve their acquisition of knowledge and skills. Apart from teaching, they have to also assess to what extent the students have learned and the areas that need further improvement, and even evaluate the curriculum to keep it dynamic and revise based on the needs assessment. It is also vital that a teacher helps the students by creating the study guide and the resource materials that will aid the students in advancing their learning [2, 6–8]. Finally, we cannot ignore the need for teachers to be good planners and should systematically plan the curriculum and organize the overall course [2].

1.2.2   Medical Teacher: Patient Care

For a common man, a doctor is someone who can cure the patient of their illnesses and sufferings. On a similar note, a medical teacher who works at a tertiary level of the healthcare delivery system is expected to extend preventive, promotive, curative, and rehabilitative care to the patients [3]. While discharging their duties, they have to be a good communicator, compassionate, and empathetic towards the sufferings of the patients and their caregivers [7]. A medical teacher is expected to offer optimal healthcare to the patients and, at the same time, utilize the opportunity of interacting with patients to teach both undergraduate and postgraduate students by maintaining a balance [3, 5].

1.2.3   Medical Teacher: Research

Teaching and research have been regarded as the two sides of the coin, and we have to acknowledge that research is an integral part of the overall growth of medicine as a profession. A medical teacher is expected to understand the importance of research and carry out the same to enhance the outcome of delivery in due course [9]. In fact, the best evidence to justify the importance of research is that it has been acknowledged as one of the primary eligibility criteria for academic promotions in Indian settings [10]. As per the recent directives of the regulatory body in India, medical teacher has to indulge in research activities that should culminate in research publications for their academic promotions [10]. Let us explore the role of research in discharging the duties of a medical teacher in the field of academics and patient care with appropriate illustrations.

1.3   Role of Research in Improving Academics

Research plays a crucial role in helping medical teachers not only sustain the basic standards in teaching but even excel in their primary role of teaching in medical institutions. For instance,

- **Meeting the needs of diversified learners:** It is not a new finding that all students learn at their own pace and have different learning styles. As a teacher, it is quite essential for them to understand the different types of learners so that they can incorporate different elements in their teaching sessions or assignments/ follow-up activities to engage all types (viz., visual learners, auditory learners, read-and-write learners, kinesthetic learners) of learners [11]. In order to understand the same, a medical teacher can carry out research to identify the distribution of different learners in the class and, based on the reported findings, change the nature of stimuli in their sessions. This will prove to be an effective strategy in facilitating learning in both classroom and beyond classroom settings and will eventually deliver encouraging results [11, 12].
- **Measuring the extent of learning:** Any teacher would want that a student who has attended their sessions should have understood the concepts and the key information passed on during the teaching-learning session. A teacher, during their session, can carry out research to get an in-depth understanding of the extent of learning by carrying out pre-test (to understand the extent of knowledge that the students have about the topic prior to the session) and post-test (to measure the change in the extent of knowledge amongst the students after the session has been taken). Based on the findings of the results, a teacher can understand the overall extent of learning among students [13].
- **Enhancing the effectiveness of sessions:** It is a fact that passive learning does not pay rich dividends and is of not much use for the students. The effectiveness of a teaching-learning session can be enhanced by ensuring the active engagement of the students in the class and the employment of interactive teaching-learning methods [14]. However, in order to ascertain the extent of benefit by the employment of an individual method can only be determined by supporting your observations with research findings [15]. For instance, a teacher can carry out research to explore the merits and the utility of problem-based learning sessions or case-based learning sessions or flipped classroom sessions. The students can be

given a semi-structured questionnaire, and they can fill the same, and the overall results can be analyzed to understand the methods that had an impact on the majority of the students. Another option is to obtain feedback from the students after the completion of each session and inquire from the students about what they liked in the class and how the session can be further improved. The teachers can analyze all the suggestions given for further improvement and incorporate them to enhance the overall effectiveness of their sessions [14, 15].

1.4   Role of Research in Improving Patient Care

Like academics, research plays an instrumental role in improving the various domains of patient care, and as a matter of fact, all the advancements in the field of patient care have been the direct outcome of research and their findings. For instance,

- **Practicing evidence-based medicine:** The need of the hour is that all medical practitioners should essentially employ evidence-based medicine in their clinical practice [16]. One of the essential aspects of the act of practicing evidence-based medicine is to do thorough research (in terms of review of literature) to identify all the literature available on the topic and various diagnostic/therapeutic options. This aspect of the review of literature helps the clinicians to select the most appropriate strategy for the management of the patients and thereby an improvement in the treatment outcome [16].
- **Improving the diagnostic abilities:** Let us consider a scenario wherein, say, 15 patients spread over a week approaches a doctor with similar kinds of symptoms and signs. Based on the common symptoms and signs, the doctor is not only able to make a common clinical diagnosis but also suggest appropriate laboratory tests for the final confirmation. Indirectly, the doctor employs the research tools in their mind and makes an evidence-based decision and thereby avoiding wastage of resources (by not asking for unwarranted tests) [17].
- **Selection of the best therapeutic modalities:** A wide range of treatment options are available for the clinicians to employ in an individual patient, but which treatment they offer to a specific patient, once again, depends upon the research findings, their earlier experience, and their knowledge/skills which they have acquired during their training period (which also originated from the research findings) [18]. For instance, the management of a patient coming with a fracture can be done by either immobilization or closed reduction, or open reduction with internal fixation. However, which treatment option will suit which patient depends on a lot of parameters (viz., site of fracture, grade of fracture, involvement of joints, affordability, etc.), and it is the clinician who takes the best decision based on their earlier experiences (evidence-based practice) [16, 18].
- **Improving the general health of the population:** At the policy-maker level, a number of decisions are being taken to improve the overall health status of the general population [19]. These decisions are not taken in isolation, and in reality,

they are based on the findings of large-scale research activities carried out in community settings [19]. For instance, the nutrition supplement that is given to under-five children in the Integrated Child Development Services Scheme for accelerating the growth of children is not a decision taken randomly. The composition of the nutritional supplement has been determined after extensive research, and it contains an adequate amount of calories and proteins for ensuring the optimal growth of the children based on their age.

- **Clinical trials:** Clinical trials play a significant role in the advancement of medicine as a branch in terms of identification of appropriate diagnostic tools for a disease/condition, selection of appropriate therapeutic strategy, and prevention of diseases (via the development of vaccines) [20]. Upon the emergence of the coronavirus disease—2019 pandemic, a significant increase in the number of clinical trials was reported across the world for identifying the drug for the treatment of the novel viral infection and for the prevention of the infection through a cost-effective vaccine [21]. As a matter of fact, it is the outcome of these extensive research activities that we have now been able to administer vaccines to the general population and subsequently reduce the incidence of acquisition of infection or the severity of the illness [21]. In addition, the findings of these clinical trials have also indicated that most of the treatment options that have been anticipated to have a significant impact on the COVID-19 infection do not carry much merit and thus have been no longer in use [22]. In short, the research findings from the clinical trials play an important role in improving the prognosis of a disease.

1.5   Research and Professional Growth

The above discussion clearly justifies the scope and utility of research in the medical field and the ways in which research can help medical teachers, senior residents, undergraduate students, and research scholars to make significant advancements in their individual professional fields [11, 16, 17]. Thus, research is a definite option for all medical teachers, and everyone should aim to indulge in research-related activities with an intention to not only improve their career prospects but also to aid in the advancement of medicine. However, the conduct of quality-assured research activities cannot be done easily, and if we really want to generate a better quality of evidence, the research work has to be carried out in large populations and, if possible, in multiple settings. This will obviously require some form of financial support, and thus all medical teachers and researchers should look for various avenues for research funding and grants.

1.6 Research Grants

In the current era, research is no longer cheap and simple, especially when we are aiming for generalizability and conduct in multiple settings. On the contrary, it is quite evident that the conduct of good research work will require financial support from the researchers so that quality can be maintained and the findings of the research will have large-scale implications. A researcher or a Medical Teacher can either apply for intramural grants (financial grants from the institution where they are working) or extramural grants (financial grants outside the institution from reputed funding agencies) [23]. However, it is a fact that none of the institutions can support all kinds of research activities in their own institution, and there arises the need to apply for extramural grants [23].

Moreover, it is a definite quality parameter in the career of a medical professional to get research funding, especially from a reputed external agency, as it is an indication that you have been involved in a work that has been duly acknowledged by the funding agency, for its quality, scope, and the impact that it will have on the health. Thus, every medical teacher and researcher should aim to get a grant/s to expand their curriculum vitae and be someone who is actively contributing to the growth of medical science. It will definitely be a challenging task, but we all can accomplish it with dedicated efforts.

However, we must realize that the process of getting grants is a competitive one, and not everyone who applies for the same will actually get it, as the funding agencies are limited. Nevertheless, we need not lose hope and continue to try to eventually receive a financial grant for research work. This is required because once we have financial support, we can actually carry out the study without compromising on its quality in a genuine manner, and it will help all the involved stakeholders. Let us consider some of the attributes for enhancing our acceptance rate for the submitted grant proposals:

- **Being aware of the funding agencies:** The first and foremost thing is to be aware of the different funding agencies, the extent of funding, the prerequisites, and the eligibility criteria for the same. This will significantly enhance your prospects as you will not miss any of the options available for getting a grant [24]. Some of the reputed funding agencies include the All India Council for Technical Education (AICTE), Council of Scientific and Industrial Research (CSIR), Indian Council of Medical Research (ICMR), Department of Biotechnology (DBT), Department of Science and Technology (DST), Indian Council of Social Science Research (ICSSR), National Science Foundation (NSF), Department of Atomic Energy (DAE), Department of Ayurveda, Yoga and Naturopathy, Unani, Siddha and Homeopathy (AYUSH), Technology Information, Forecasting and Assessment Council (TIFAC), Indian National Science Academy (INSA), Campus France, CAPES (Brazilian Federal Agency for the Support and Evaluation of Graduate Education), IIE: The Power of International Education, CNPq—National Council for Scientific and Technological Development, COST—European Cooperation in

Science & Technology, DAAD—In-Country/In-Region Program in Developing Countries, etc.

- **Stating the goal of the project and the need for the same:** It is quite essential that the research project for which the research grant has been applied is something that is important from the public health perspective. You should clearly justify the goal of the project, how you will go ahead with the task (adopted procedures), the expected outcomes of your project, and eventually, the gaps that will be addressed in the research process [23].
- **The novelty of the research project:** Almost all extramural funding agencies look forward to funding a research project that is novel, and thus all the investigators should aim to explore a new dimension through their research. This will not only cast a good impact on the funding agency but will also aid in the advancement of science [24].
- **Writing style:** The grant proposal has to be written keeping in mind the interest of the reviewers who will be evaluating the proposal. It should be simple yet scientifically written, specific attention should be given to the required heading, and a clear explanation of budgeting also should be given [24, 25].
- **Principal Investigator and the Team:** Any funding agency will definitely give consideration to the profile of the principal investigator and other co-investigators. It is always good to do some kind of work in the field in which you are applying for funding so that the funding agency can look for your contribution and establish the veracity of the proposal. Further, considering that good quality research work cannot be carried out by a single person, it is ideal to apply for a grant along with a team comprising of qualified professionals, with their roles and responsibilities clearly defined. This will be another step in enhancing the acceptance rate of your grant proposal [23–25].

1.7   Conclusion

To conclude, a medical teacher is expected to excel in the field of teaching, patient care, research, and administration. Research is one of the key domains that will also aid a Medical Teacher or a Researcher in performing better in the domains of teaching, patient care, and administration. However, the conduction of quality-assured research work will essentially require financial support in the form of research grants, and that is what all the researchers should aim for and accordingly work in the same direction.

Case Scenario
1. A postgraduate student from the department of pediatrics who had a passion for teaching joined a medical college upon completion of his postgraduation. Soon he realized that medical teacher has to discharge multiple roles other than teaching to not only benefit themselves but also the medical students and the patients. Enumerate the various roles of a medical teacher.

References

1. Nawabi S, Shaikh SS, Javed MQ, Riaz A. Faculty's perception of their role as a medical teacher at Qassim University, Saudi Arabia. Cureus. 2020;12(7):e9095.
2. Harden RM, Crosby JO. AMEE Guide No. 20—the good teacher is more than a lecturer—the twelve roles of the teacher. Med Teach. 2000;22:334–47.
3. van den Berg JW, Verberg CPM, Scherpbier AJJA, Jaarsma ADC, Arah OA, Lombarts KMJMH. Faculty's work engagement in patient care: impact on job crafting of the teacher tasks. BMC Med Educ. 2018;18(1):312.
4. Schriner C, Deckelman S, Kubat MA, Lenkay J, Nims L, Sullivan D. Collaboration of nursing faculty and college administration in creating organizational change. Nurs Educ Perspect. 2010;31(6):381–6.
5. Ramani S. Twelve tips to promote excellence in medical teaching. Med Teach. 2006;28:19–23.
6. Amey L, Donald KJ, Teodorczuk A. Teaching clinical reasoning to medical students. Br J Hosp Med (Lond). 2017;78(7):399–401.
7. Modi JN, Anshu GP, Singh T. Teaching and assessing professionalism in the Indian context. Indian Pediatr. 2014;51(11):881–8.
8. Paritakul P, Wongwandee M, Tantitemit T, Pumipichet S, Dennick R. Level of confidence in the 12 roles of a medical teacher. A descriptive study at Faculty of Medicine, Srinakharinwirot University, Thailand. J Med Assoc Thai. 2015;98(Suppl 10):S38–44.
9. Mazzer PA, Melroe LB. Beyond the single course: teaching research throughout the curriculum. Adv Physiol Educ. 2019;43(2):168–71.
10. Shrivastava SR, Shrivastava PS. Critiquing the revised minimum qualifications for promotion of medical teachers in India. Natl Med J India. 2020;33(5):316–8.
11. Bhalli MA, Khan IA, Sattar A. Learning style of medical students and its correlation with preferred teaching methodologies and academic achievement. J Ayub Med Coll Abbottabad. 2015;27(4):837–42.
12. Ojeh N, Sobers-Grannum N, Gaur U, Udupa A, Majumder MAA. Learning style preferences: a study of pre-clinical medical students in Barbados. J Adv Med Educ Prof. 2017;5(4):185–94.
13. Thai TTN, Pham TT, Nguyen KT, Nguyen PM, Derese A. Can a family medicine rotation improve medical students' knowledge, skills and attitude towards primary care in Vietnam? A pre-test–post-test comparison and qualitative survey. Trop Med Int Health. 2020;25(2):264–75.
14. Begum J, Ali SI, Panda M. Introduction of interactive teaching for undergraduate students in community medicine. Indian J Community Med. 2020;45(1):72–6.
15. Kuchynska IO, Palamar BI, Ilashchuk TO, Bobkovych KO, Davydova NV, Polishchuk SV. Innovative and interactive teaching methods as a means of optimizing the educational process of higher medical education. Wiad Lek. 2019;72(11 cz 1):2149–54.
16. Nicholson J, Kalet A, van der Vleuten C, de Bruin A. Understanding medical student evidence-based medicine information seeking in an authentic clinical simulation. J Med Libr Assoc. 2020;108(2):219–28.
17. Campagnolo AM, Priston J, Thoen RH, Medeiros T, Assunção AR. Laryngopharyngeal reflux: diagnosis, treatment, and latest research. Int Arch Otorhinolaryngol. 2014;18(2):184–91.
18. Wu ZQ, Zeng DL, Yao JL, Bian YY, Gu YT, Meng ZL, et al. Research progress on diagnosis and treatment of chronic osteomyelitis. Chin Med Sci J. 2019;34(3):211–20.
19. Howley NL, Hunt H. Every school healthy: policy, research, and action. J Sch Health. 2020;90 (12):903–6.
20. Livhits MJ, Zhu CY, Kuo EJ, Nguyen DT, Kim J, Tseng CH, et al. Effectiveness of molecular testing techniques for diagnosis of indeterminate thyroid nodules: a randomized clinical trial. JAMA Oncol. 2021;7(1):70–7.
21. Janiaud P, Axfors C, Van't Hooft J, Saccilotto R, Agarwal A, Appenzeller-Herzog C, et al. The worldwide clinical trial research response to the COVID-19 pandemic—the first 100 days. F1000Res. 2020;9:1193.

22. Li L, Zhang W, Hu Y, Tong X, Zheng S, Yang J, et al. Effect of convalescent plasma therapy on time to clinical improvement in patients with severe and life-threatening COVID-19: a randomized clinical trial. JAMA. 2020;324(5):460–70.
23. Harper L, Castagnetti M, Herbst K, Bagli D, Kaefer M, Beckers G, et al. How to apply for a research grant: 10 tips and tricks. J Pediatr Urol. 2018;14(5):453–4.
24. Jones HP, McGee R, Weber-Main AM, Buchwald DS, Manson SM, Vishwanatha JK, et al. Enhancing research careers: an example of a US national diversity-focused, grant-writing training and coaching experiment. BMC Proc. 2017;11(Suppl 12):16.
25. Blanco MA, Lee MY. Twelve tips for writing educational research grant proposals. Med Teach. 2012;34(6):450–3.

What Is a Grant? How to Prepare a Grant Proposal Application

Vikram Kate, R. Kalayarasan, and Sathasivam Sureshkumar

By failing to prepare, you are preparing to fail

Benjamin Franklin

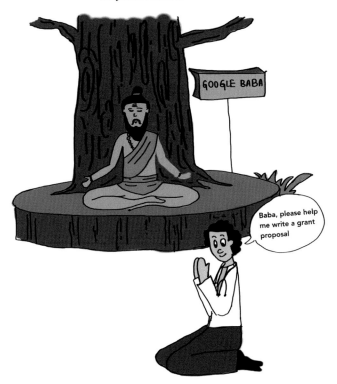

What is a grant how to prepare for writing a grant proposal application

V. Kate (✉)
Department of General and Gastrointestinal surgery, Jawaharlal Institute of Postgraduate Medical Education and Research (JIPMER), Pondicherry, India

R. Kalayarasan
Department of Surgical Gastroenterology, Jawaharlal Institute of Post-Graduate Medical Education and Research (JIPMER), Pondicherry, India

© The Author(s), under exclusive license to Springer Nature Singapore Pte Ltd. 2023
S. C. Parija, V. Kate (eds.), *Grant writing for medical and healthcare professionals*,
https://doi.org/10.1007/978-981-19-7018-4_2

13

Objectives
- To understand what a grant is.
- Importance of obtaining a grant.
- How to prepare a grant application.
- Understand the differences in writing the grant proposal from other research proposals.

2.1   What is a Grant?

The very reason modern medicine is accepted and adapted worldwide is that the current medical science is built on evidence-based medicine. The evidence, of course, is created and established by well-structured research works. A quality research outcome requires a well-established research setup and the resources which mandate reasonable funding. The funding covers the expenses of the research equipment, manpower, and compensation for the time spent on the research by the researcher and the staff [1, 2]. The funding may be acquired from the institute of the researcher or funding organizations. This funding provided for conducting research work is commonly referred to as a research grant. Conventionally, the financial assistance for the research and the grant is allotted competitively, especially when acquired from the funding organizations.

Considering the limited budget allocation for the research assistance and a large number of funding requests by the researchers, the grants are awarded only to a small proportion of the grant applicants [1–3]. Since there is a rigorous reviewing process and scrutiny involved in providing the research funding, receiving the research grant indicates that the grant proposal is superior to others in quality, feasibility with a more desirable output, and the completion of the research in time. A grant proposal writing also provides the researcher an opportunity to conceptualize the hypothesis and write in detail the research framework mentioning every finer detail and thus making a roadmap for carrying out the study [1]. This makes the research protocol better, increases the probability of completing the research, and paves the way for future direction. Considering the competitive atmosphere for obtaining the grant and the importance of the research grant in carrying the high impact research, it is of paramount importance for the young researcher to master the technique of writing the grant proposal, which has now become a fundamental requisite for career progression in the academic medical field [4].

S. Sureshkumar
Department of Surgery, Jawaharlal Institute of Post-Graduate Medical Education and Research (JIPMER), Pondicherry, India

2.2   Types of Grants in Academic Medical Institutions

Grants can be intramural, where the researcher's institute or the agency funds the project, which is usually for smaller projects which need limited funding for a period of 2–3 years [1, 5]. As a young faculty or the researcher need to establish their area of interest, focus, and competence in their research work, these intramural grants are provided in their early career, usually within 3–5 years after joining. This is also called career development grants, as it helps the young faculty to grow to a level to get extramural funding in their field of interest [1, 5, 6]. The researcher is expected to acquire significant extramural grants after the initial assistance from intramural grants to continue or progress in their research field. Extramural grants are also called project grants as they, in general, are provided for a specified research project. The governmental or non-governmental organizations provide extramural grants with a particular objective in the medical field. The funding sources may be non-profit governmental or non-profit or for-profit non-governmental private organizations, including industries and charity groups [7].

2.3   Importance of Obtaining a Grant

A faculty working in an academic medical institution is expected to achieve specified targets in a multidimensional platform, including teaching, services, and research, to get the academic promotion and ascending credentials for progress. Though the teaching and services offered by the faculty are given due consideration in the career progression, the more measurable and achievable targets that most medical institutions expect from the faculty are research grants and publications in high-impact journals [8]. The quality of the publication is generally measured by the impact factor of the journal, and though the studies have shown that the publication in high impact factor journals is not an appropriate measure of the quality of the research work, the majority of the organizations consider a number of publications in high impact factor journals as an essential measure for the academic promotions [9].

A good-quality publication can happen from a good-quality research work that requires substantial funding in most instances. Studies have shown that the average age of receiving independent funding has gone up from 38 in 1980 to 40–45 in 2013 [10]. Though the higher number of grant applications and reduced budget for governmental funding organizations can be attributed to this change, the poorly written incomplete grant application which lacks clarity on the concept and method has been shown as one of the important factors for not obtaining research grant by many faculties. Also, the grant proposal writing has not been given enough importance in the academic curricula in the graduate programs where the young researcher starts their academic career [11]. Writing a successful grant application requires training, adequate time, and perseverance. Some educational institutions aid in writing grant proposals by offering editorial assistance, training sessions, and internal review mechanism. Considering the policy adopted by most academic medical institutions for career advancement and promotion, it is of paramount importance for young faculty and researchers to read and train themselves in writing a successful grant application. The successful funding record also increases the chance of obtaining further research funding for conducting more advanced projects.

2.4   How to Prepare for Writing a Grant Proposal Application

Developing a research idea is the first preparatory step in writing a grant proposal application (Fig. 2.1). In the most common scenario, the researcher develops a research idea based on the unmet clinical needs and then applies for a grant from the appropriate organization instead of inventing a research topic for funding. A typical example is the Science and Engineering Research Board invites applications for a core research grant every year during a specified period. The researcher applies during the window period of the grant application. Occasionally scientific bodies invite grant research proposals on a particular topic. Indian Council of Medical Research (ICMR) inviting research proposal related to severe acute respiratory syndrome coronavirus 2 (SARS-CoV-2) during the COVID-19 pandemic is an example of topic-specific grant proposals initiated by the research organizations. The researcher with novel ideas can apply for it. A brief overview of the preparation required for a successful grant application is enumerated below.

- Think of yourself as a project reviewer and ask the following questions about your research idea. Does the study have merit, and what is the potential impact? Developmental work of the already done research project (incremental research) or a routine application of known techniques (low impact research) does not incite interest among the reviewers and grant agency. The researcher should do an extensive literature review to ensure that the proposed research topic is novel.
- Always discuss your research ideas with colleagues and mentors. We might often think our research topic is the most creative, but it may be otherwise. It is essential to come out of the comfort zone and be open to suggestions from peers and mentors that will realistically improve the research proposal. The inputs from successful grant applicants, especially when for the same funding agency, can improve the proposal significantly by providing the necessary important tips necessary for success.
- The research topic should be creative and exciting for you and the reviewing agency. The grant agency will find your research idea interesting if it falls in their thrust areas of research. Identify the funding agency based on the type of research grant required for your study. You can go through the grant organization's website or contact the program officer, share your research idea, and get their input on whether the proposed research falls in their priority areas. Networking with program officers through conferences and professional meetings would help understand what the funding agencies are looking for in the grant proposal. Also, you should contact people who have written successful grant applications and received a grant from the agency to understand what it took to receive funds.

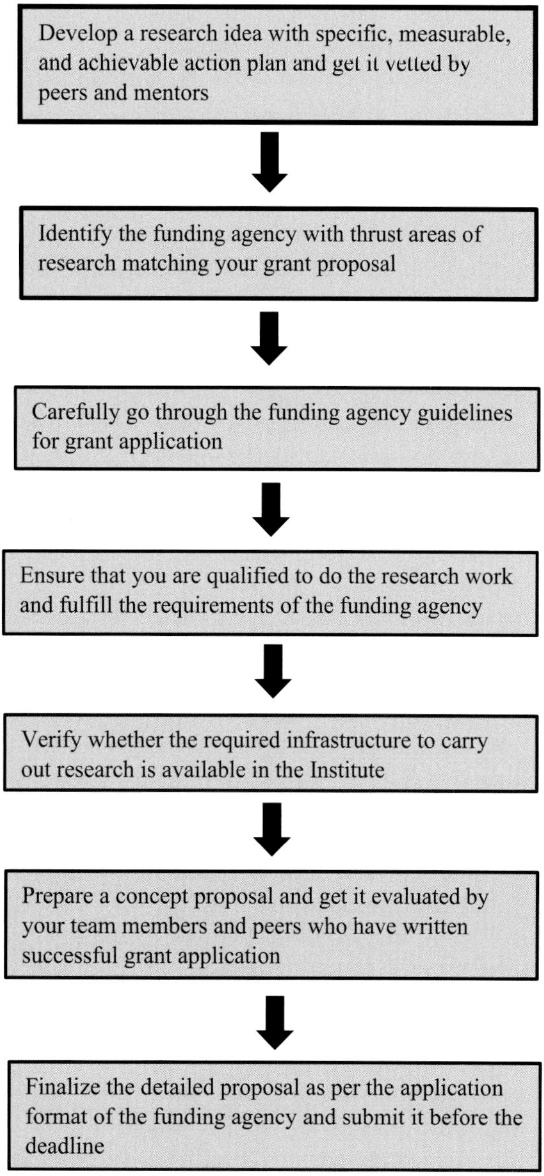

Fig. 2.1 Preparatory steps for writing a grant proposal application

Develop a research idea with specific, measurable, and achievable action plan and get it vetted by peers and mentors

Identify the funding agency with thrust areas of research matching your grant proposal

Carefully go through the funding agency guidelines for grant application

Ensure that you are qualified to do the research work and fulfill the requirements of the funding agency

Verify whether the required infrastructure to carry out research is available in the Institute

Prepare a concept proposal and get it evaluated by your team members and peers who have written successful grant application

Finalize the detailed proposal as per the application format of the funding agency and submit it before the deadline

- Form an interdisciplinary team for your research proposal. Think big and cross the boundaries of your department, institution, and country, as in the current world, it is always better to do superior work with collaboration.
- Funding agencies give priority to multi-institutional collaboration projects. While doing collaborative research, it is crucial to identify the team members who would add value and strength to your project to make the collaboration meaningful.

Collaborators should have complementary expertise, and it is necessary to obtain a letter of support from collaborators.

- Understand the differences in writing the grant proposal from other research proposals. As funding agencies are often government organizations that use public money for the grant, it is essential to highlight how your research proposal fits the nation's health care needs. Write a responsive proposal keeping in mind the requirements of the funding agency. Parse the call for proposal and ensure that you have addressed all the requirements. Follow the exact format of the application with a clear statement of the benefits and significance of your research in the abstract, introduction, and conclusions. Highlight why your research should be considered a priority and the expected impact of knowledge and advancement generated from your study. Avoid fishing expeditions and provide a strong rationale for the research work. The research proposal should demonstrate innovation and significance within its field of study. It should have a well-defined research plan and be presented in a language that the reviewers can easily understand, even if they are not subject experts.

- Include a clear schedule and describe the deliverables of your research. As with any research proposal, grant proposal outcomes should be specific, measurable, achievable, realistic, and timely (SMART). Your grant proposal should demonstrate that project can be completed in a stipulated period as funding agencies do not want to stretch the timelines.

- Create an appropriate budget plan and justify the budget expenditures so that the funding agency finds it realistic. Review the guidelines from the funding agency and determine the heads required for budgeting. Develop and format the budget by calculating the costs required under each head. Provide adequate justification for various budget heads. Ensure that budget heads match the funding agency guidelines. While most organizations provide a grant for manpower, consumables, and travel-related to research, some funding agencies also support equipment procurement, provide compensation for research participants, and cover research-related publication costs. It is essential to understand that the review process and acceptance of the grant application are primarily determined by the scientific content of the proposal and are not budget-oriented unless the proposed budget is grossly out of range and beyond the scope of the funding agencies. Hence, even a small budget grant application can get rejected if the application is not well written.

- The grant proposal should demonstrate that the investigators are qualified to do the study as the funding agencies want to ensure that the grant is not wasted. Prepare a good curriculum vitae (CV) highlighting your research work and research publications. The CV should demonstrate your expertise in proposed research by highlighting your past accomplishments. It should also highlight the successfully completed grant-related projects leading to good publications.

- Ensure that the research environment in the institute is conducive to doing the proposed research. The feasibility of research work in your setup is an essential criterion for selection by the funding agencies. Prepare a range of supporting materials highlighting the research infrastructure in your institute. Some agencies also need a letter of support from the institute to utilize the facilities for the project.

- Some funding agencies will invite concept proposals in the initial phase and request detailed proposals from the selected participants with novel ideas for the final decision. Even if the funding agency does not ask for a concept proposal, it is always a good practice to prepare a concept proposal with a title, introduction (approximately 300 words), novelty (approximately 200 words), applicability (approximately 200 words), short- and long-term objectives, description of the project (1000 words), why the project is a priority and its expected impact on the general population.

- Set a timeline and give yourself sufficient time to write the grant proposal rather than writing a project close to the deadline. The calendar for grant applications is often fixed for funding agencies, and the researcher should plan accordingly. Complete the proposal at least 3 weeks before the deadline so that you can get feedback from the team and peers or mentors. Show the research proposal to the peer who knows your area of work well and to the peer who is not a specialist in your area, as the reviewers may not always be subject experts.

- Grant writing could be a painful process and prepare for rejections as the funds are limited and proposals keep increasing every year. Common reasons for rejection are too ambitious research proposal with unfocussed aims and objectives, lack of compelling rationale, and little demonstration of institutional support or resources to accomplish the research project. Review the comments carefully and revise your proposal if the project is rejected. The chance of success improves with the second or third submission.

Although the grant writing process may seem daunting, it is a skill that every researcher should master to have a successful academic career. Preparatory steps highlighted in the chapter will guide the researcher in writing a successful grant application.

2.5   Conclusion

A quality research outcome requires a well-established research setup and the resources which mandate reasonable funding. A better-quality publication can only originate from a high-impact research work that requires substantial funding in a required time frame. Since there is a rigorous reviewing process and scrutiny involved in providing the research funding, receiving the research grant indicates the higher quality of the research and the feasibility of the completion of the research and the resultant outcome. Hence, grant proposal writing has become an essential skill that all researchers need to master. As with any research proposal, grant proposal outcomes should be specific, measurable, achievable, realistic, and timely (SMART). Developing a research idea, including a clear budget plan, ensuring a conducive research environment in the institute, and setting up a timeline for completing the grant application are the important parts of writing the grant proposal.

Case Scenarios

1. Indian Council of Medical Research (ICMR) had invited researchers to submit research grant proposals on innovative treatment options for gastrointestinal cancers. You are planning to write a grant proposal. How would you ensure that your grant application is successful?
   Will you plan it as a single institution or multi-institutional project?
2. A young assistant professor wants to establish his area of interest and do focused research work.
   What would be the better option for him to receive a grant?
   What are the limiting factors for him to obtain the extramural research grant?
   What are the strategies for writing a successful grant proposal?

References

1. Inouye SK, Fiellin DA. An evidence-based guide to writing grant proposals for clinical research. Ann Intern Med. 2005;142(4):274–82. https://doi.org/10.7326/0003-4819-142-4-200502150-00009.
2. Gholipour A, Lee EY, Warfield SK. The anatomy and art of writing a successful grant application: a practical step-by-step approach. Pediatr Radiol. 2014;44(12):1512–7. https://doi.org/10.1007/s00247-014-3051-8.
3. Brownson RC, Colditz GA, Dobbins M, Emmons KM, Kerner JF, Padek M, Proctor EK, Stange KC. Concocting that magic elixir: successful grant application writing in dissemination and implementation research. Clin Transl Sci. 2015;8(6):710–6. https://doi.org/10.1111/cts.12356.
4. Schimanski LA, Alperin JP. The evaluation of scholarship in academic promotion and tenure processes: past, present, and future. F1000Res. 2018;7:1605. https://doi.org/10.12688/f1000research.16493.1.
5. Liu JC, Pynnonen MA, St John M, Rosenthal EL, Couch ME, Schmalbach CE. Grant-writing pearls and pitfalls: maximizing funding opportunities. Otolaryngol Head Neck Surg. 2016;154(2):226–32. https://doi.org/10.1177/0194599815620174.
6. Mughal A, Wahlberg KJ, Li Z, Flyer JN, Olson NC, Cushman M. Impact of an institutional grant award on early career investigator applicants and peer reviewers. Res Pract Thromb Haemost. 2021;5(5):e12555. https://doi.org/10.1002/rth2.12555.
7. Urrutia R. Academic skills: a concise guide to grant writing. Pancreatology. 2007;7(4):307–10. https://doi.org/10.1159/000106761.
8. Mbuagbaw L, Anderson LN, Lokker C, Thabane L. Advice for junior faculty regarding academic promotion: what not to worry about, and what to worry about. J Multidiscip Healthc. 2020;13:117–22. https://doi.org/10.2147/JMDH.S240056.
9. McKiernan EC, Schimanski LA, Nieves CM, Matthias L, Niles MT, Alperin JP. Use of the Journal Impact Factor in academic review, promotion, and tenure evaluations. Elife. 2019;8:e47338.
10. Daniels RJ. A generation at risk: young investigators and the future of the biomedical workforce. Proc Natl Acad Sci. 2015;112(2):313–8.
11. Dumanis SB, Ullrich L, Washington PM, Forcelli PA. It's money! Real-world grant experience through a student-run, peer-reviewed program. CBE Life Sci Educ. 2013;12(3):419–28.

Funders' Perspective: What the Funding Body Expects from Researchers?

3

Manju Rahi, Sachin Sharma, and Bhawna Yadav

Meeting expectations is good. Exceeding expectations is better

Ron Kaufman

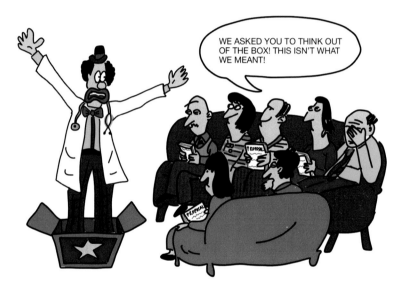

Funders perspective

Objectives
- To highlight the key points to consider while conceptualizing and writing a grant application.

M. Rahi (✉) · S. Sharma · B. Yadav
Indian Council of Medical Research, New Delhi, India

S. C. Parija, V. Kate (eds.), *Grant writing for medical and healthcare professionals*,
https://doi.org/10.1007/978-981-19-7018-4_3

Writing is the essential core skill for every researcher who wishes to procure a research grant. This is one of the ways that one can communicate their work or plans to their peers, reviewers, or target audience. Nearly every researcher or scientist needs to write grants and gain funding in order to carry out their research. In today's competitive environment, all the institutions/universities assess the performance of their scientific staff based on the successful funding achieved in addition to other parameters. Many institutes during recruitment even consider the in-hand grants or a successful track record of completed projects as well as the potential of the applicants to obtain funding and prefer such candidates and justifiably so. As such, grant writing is a skill that every researcher has to develop. However, it does not just stop here. Winning grant writing is the ultimate target, and successful execution with the dissemination of results in high-quality journals and conferences is the logical conclusion. The aim of this chapter is to present the funder's/sponsors perspective while assessing the grant applications and providing the prospective grant writers with key considerations while planning their grant application.

3.1   Funding Agencies are Looking for Good Proposals—They Want to Fund Research

While there are several funding agencies (government and private) and organizations to fund good work [1], most researchers complain about the high rejection rates of grant applications. The first and foremost thing to remember is that the funding agencies are there to support and fund research, not to reject or discourage research. They really want to support good and impactful proposals which are in line with their mission, and this is one of the parameters of their success. However, they also want value for their money. Most funding agencies work with public money, and every funded project must be justifiable. A proposal needs to stand out from the rest of the proposals to gather the interest of the sponsor. Also, even if the proposal is excellent, if it is not presented well, it may get rejected.

There can be two types of funding calls, namely a broad/general funding call with the theme chosen by the grant applicant, i.e., "investigator driven" (e.g., a call for funding in basic sciences); or calls for very specific themes, i.e., "theme-driven," decided by the funding program {e.g., ICMR,'s Malaria Elimination Research Alliance-India (MERA-India) program} calling for proposals on innovative vector control tools to support malaria elimination. The proposed research plan should be in line with the vision and mission of the funding agency. This does not mean that the grant applicant should change his/her basic proposed idea to align with the goals of the funding agency. The right selection is the fundamental concept here, and the researcher should not try to "fit" or "adjust" his research work (proposed and current) to the theme of the call given for proposals. Instead, the researcher should first think about their research plan and then look for the funding agencies that are supporting such research goals [2]. Each of the funding agencies have specific research priorities, and while they are supporting the researchers working in those directions, the researchers are equally important for them to achieve their strategic goals, and as such both are interdependent on each other for their success.

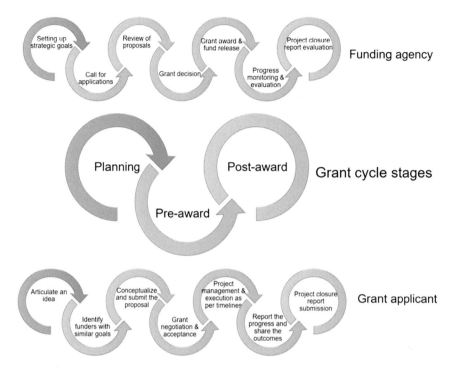

Fig. 3.1 The grant cycle stages—The grant cycle can be divided into planning, pre-award, and post-award stages, with defined roles for the funding agencies as well as the grant applicants during each stage

3.2   Funding Agencies Have Different Grant Cycles—Keep a Track of Them

Different funding agencies have different grant cycles (Fig. 3.1) and timelines as per their mandate. The applicant should keep a track of the grant cycles of the different funders and should start preparing their applications accordingly. It is advisable that researchers should not wait for the announcement of the call for preparing their applications. It is always better to plan the grant application well in advance. Most of the funding bodies ask for preliminary work and results thereof to be reported in the proposal. Therefore, the intervening period between the two calls should be used for generating that preliminary data as a precursor to the proposed research work.

It is suggested to be in communication with the funding agencies at every stage of the grant cycle. With most of the funding bodies, the applications and the review processes are online and thus communication has become easier and quicker. In fact, in certain cases, it is advisable to discuss the research idea with the funders beforehand to see if it aligns with their goals.

3.3   Write the Application in the Format That the Funder Wants to Read—Keep the Writing Simple and Organized

Just as most of the journals have similar sections but have different format guidelines, similarly, most of the grant applications also require almost similar information, but in a format specified by the funding agency, to ensure uniformity across the applications received. Even if the proposal is excellent in all aspects, if it does not adhere to the specified format, it will be returned for revision or may even be immediately rejected without any consideration. Hence, compliance with the prescribed guidelines (sections, word limit, font size, review of literature, proposed budget format, and others) enhances the chances of the application being viewed favorably. The guidelines may change from time to time, so it is important to refer to the latest set of information. In case of doubt, the applicants should communicate to the funding agency and ensure that they abide by the most recent guidelines.

Many times applicants try to fit in a lot of information and use methods such as reducing the margin size or font size. Some applicants try to emphasize specific information using a combination of formatting such as making the text bold, italicizing and underlining. The write-up in this fashion can be distracting for the reviewer from the main study, and the details may be lost [3]. Not following the instructions gives an impression of a casual attitude and may go against the applicant. The reviewers are also busy with their science and their own grants and projects and, most of the time, are not paid to review the applications; they do it as an honorary service to the scientific community. As such, you should make every effort to make it easier for the reviewer to understand your proposal such that they do not have to search for the information in the application.

The title of the proposal should indicate the type of study, the main proposed work, and the settings of the study. It should not be too lengthy but should capture all essential elements. The sections and sub-sections should be organized and connected logically. The headings should be clear and precise to indicate the contents of the paragraphs. Numbering the headings and sub-headings helps the reviewers to navigate easily through the application.

The proposals should not be too wordy. Give the key messages in a concise and to the point manner. Long sentences and paragraphs should be avoided. Providing the information as bullet points and use of figures, graphics, flowcharts, etc., wherever possible, makes the reading more lucid [4]. An abstract, in the beginning or as per the format of the application, is the backbone of the proposal and is very helpful for the reviewers to understand the proposed work.

The reviewing panel will have experts from diverse research backgrounds. The proposal should be written for the entire reviewing panel in such a way that even a non-specialist can understand the problem and your proposed solution. It helps to take the opinions of the colleagues in the same and different fields while maintaining confidentiality. Spelling mistakes and grammatical errors should be minimized.

3.4   Provide Clear Objectives of the Study

This is an extremely important section of the proposal. The objectives of the proposed work should be clearly articulated. They should be realistic, measurable, achievable, and fit well within the duration of the proposed work [5]. They should be in line with the overall theme as wanted by the funding body.

3.5   Present the Latest Scenario in the Proposed Field of Research—and Why Your Research Should be Funded Over Others

A thorough and up-to-date review of literature should be carried out, citing the significant and important studies along with facts and figures. The review should be in line with the proposed work highlighting scientific work carried out so far and gaps in the current understanding of how the proposed work can be a step towards filling that gap. It is advised to have a neutral tone while citing others' work, without expressing any bias for or against any specific group (which could be the work of the reviewer itself or the reviewer's collaborating/competing group). The highlight of the application should be the proposed work and how it will take the existing knowledge ahead. Therefore, the strengths and novelty of the proposed research as compared to the other studies should be very clear. It is also essential to highlight the applicant's experience and expertise, which make him/her the best candidate to drive the proposed research. This does not mean that the applicant (early career researcher) must have a background in the proposed work. Coming out from the comfort zone and entering into a new field may be considered a bold step and thus a bonus point. However, continuing in the same field has its own advantages, like providing a proven track record and preliminary data.

3.6   Provide Preliminary Data if Possible

It is always a plus point to provide preliminary data or scoping research. This establishes credibility and confidence in the proposed plan and the applicant [6]. This is particularly helpful when the applicant is new to the proposed area of research. Even if the preliminary data pertains to only a specific section of the application, it convinces the reviewers of the seriousness of the applicant to pursue the proposed research and also helps to validate the approach.

3.7   Provide Clear Methodology—Show That You Know What to Do and How to Do

While describing the methodology, it is very important that the most appropriate and the latest methods in the field are chosen. The methods proposed should be able to achieve the specific objectives and outputs. It should be stated if the instruments for the method execution are available with the grant applicant, accessible in other groups or institutions, or will have to be purchased.

The sample source, as applicable, should be precisely indicated. For example, if an animal or human/clinical samples would be involved, the source and collaborations should be provided. It should be mentioned if the samples would be available year-round or seasonally, and the methodology should be devised according to this. In the case of microbial strains, it should be mentioned if the material transfer agreements (MTAs) are already in place or if there is a collaborator willing to provide the strains. The sample size should be statistically calculated using power calculation, and a random number should not be quoted [7].

If the research involves some ethical concerns, it is important to mention the ways that will be adopted to address that concern. For any sensitive issues, approval from the concerned organization/authorities would help convince the reviewers that the research will not face any roadblocks during execution. For animal studies, or research involving human subjects, ethical clearance from the institutional ethical committee or appropriate advisor/regulatory board should have been granted or should be in the process of consideration to demonstrate that the samples/specimen would be available immediately for the proposed study.

If there are collaborators and partners in the study from other groups or institutions, their roles, responsibility, and assigned work should be clearly mentioned.

It is also essential to describe the anticipated challenges during the course of the study and the ways to tackle those challenges. A backup plan or an alternative approach in case the primary screening or an experiment fails is expected by the reviewers as it helps to convince them that the study will not be stalled in such scenarios.

3.8   Show the Plan for Data Collection, Analysis, and Sharing

A clear strategy should be given for the data acquisition, storage, and management and for data sharing and availability. The computational resources with the applicant or the host institution should be provided. The software for data analysis (free or licensed) should be indicated. It should be mentioned if the applicant has the technical know-how and expertise for the data analysis and statistical significance or if there is a collaborator for such analyses. These details strengthen your application and help assure the reviewers of a well-thought data organization plan.

3.9   Provide Realistic Timelines and Goals

It is very important to provide realistic timelines and goals according to the duration quoted for the proposed work and the funding requested. Both overambitious and under-delivery of goals would lead to negative scores. A reasonable plan with achievable goals within the funding timeline and with the available or requested resources should be proposed.

A Gantt chart with the project schedule, including the activities like hiring and training the staff, procurement of chemicals and instruments, experimental work, data collection, and analysis, as well as the packaging of the final output and dissemination, should be provided. This helps to convince the reviewers that the applicant has thoroughly planned for the entire funding period and would be able to successfully manage and work towards the mentioned goals. The most common comments from the reviewers are—the "Overambitious" proposal which does not seem realistic or "very less" work proposed in the given duration. Remember shooting for the moon does not always work. Therefore, well-balanced goals always carry an advantage.

3.10   State the Impact of the Study

The proposal should describe the short-term as well as the long-term impacts of the proposed research. The plan should suggest how it will advance the understanding in the field. The target population, geographical area, or the proposed influence on the policies should be clearly stated. The sustainability of the project is also important, for example, how the study will continue after this specific funding is over. The funders would prefer studies that would be of broad interest and are likely to sustain interest and support from different agencies and sponsors. The proposed plan for disseminating the output should also be stated.

3.11   Ask the Funders for What you Need—Know How Much they can Give

It is very crucial to ask for funding for the right resources and in the right amount. While proposing the budget, it should be honest and realistic. The maximum limit of the funding agency should be kept in mind, and the budget should be accordingly prepared. The specific support from the host institution should be highlighted, which shows the willingness of the host institution. An appropriate justification should be provided for each type of expense expected [1].

3.12   Public Outreach Activities

All the funding agencies expect transparency and accountability for the appropriate use of funds. Public outreach activities are becoming an important component of the research plans. The researchers and scientists are obliged to share their research outputs and the tools generated with the scientific as well as general communities. And as such, the application should also highlight the ways that such activities would be carried out [2]. This makes a favorable impression on the reviewers, and for many funding agencies, this is now an integral part of the applications. After all, this is taxpayer's money, and everyone with or without scientific background has the right to know the significance of the output of the study. The method and way to be adopted should be corroborated with the line of work. The audience would be different from a public health study with operational/implementation components (public health experts, program managers, community) than from a study on basic sciences (peers, students, scholars). Also, school/college students can be invited to visit the lab, with a description of the scientific journey of the study and investigator as an inspiration for the younger generation.

3.13   Cite Appropriate References

Any fact should be supported by an appropriate reference. However, do not use excessive references for every sentence [3]. The cited papers should be appropriate and not controversial. Do not cite a review that refers to the original work; the original study should be cited. Usually, the referencing style is indicated in the funding agency's guidelines for application preparation.

3.14   Check for Plagiarism Score

Before submitting the application, the applicant should run it on the plagiarism detection software. Sometimes the funding agencies provide an acceptable plagiarism score, and accordingly, the application should be corrected.

3.15   Choose the Right Co-investigators and Collaborators

The right collaborators or co-investigators who can complement the applicant and fulfill the lack of experience/skill of the applicant for a specific aspect of the study are essential [6]. The nature of collaboration should be clearly stated, for example, if the role of the collaborator is to provide samples or access to instruments or technical expertise. It is important to justify the role, expertise, and contribution of each of the team members at each level: mentor, co-investigator, collaborator, etc.

3.16   Choose the Right Host Institution

The choice of the host institution is of utmost importance. The applicant should see if the goals of the host institution align with the proposed research objectives. The reviewers assess if the host institution has the capacity to successfully manage grants and projects. The host institution's support in the form of providing infrastructure, appropriate lab space, resources, or career development support to the young applicant or to the PhD students and technical staff enrolled in the project are all important considerations for the reviewers to determine the suitability of the host institution. It is also important that the host institution accepts the funding agency's terms and conditions. For example, different funders give a different percentage of grants to the host institution as overhead charges. The host institution has to accept the amount allotted, and there cannot be any negotiations on this.

3.17   Provide Genuine Letters of Support

Strong and genuine letters of support from the host organization, as well as mentors or collaborators, play a key role in the reviewers' assessment of the applicant's capabilities and commitment [4]. Remember that the reviewers would have seen hundreds of letters of support and can thus clearly distinguish between a general, copy-paste letter and a specific letter of support specific for the applicant and the proposed study. This is interlinked with the above paragraph, "choose the right host institution." If the host institution is genuinely interested in hosting you, you will definitely get a strong letter(s) of support.

3.18   Learn from the Rejections—Try Again

Even the most experienced and senior researchers have faced grant rejections at some point of time in their careers. Do not get disappointed. In case the application is rejected, do not submit a fresh application without understanding the cause of rejection [4]. At times it can be simply because the applicant did not adhere to the funder's guidelines. Or it could be that a specific section was not presented, and hence it was not clear to the reviewers. Many times the funders share feedback for the applications. Instead of becoming critical and cynical, take the comments of the funding organization constructively and use these comments as a stepping stone for making the study better. Get in touch with the funders, seriously work on the feedback and try to understand how the application can be improved for a favorable review, they are always happy to help. If invited for re-submission, address all the concerns of the funders within the given time frame. Maintain your relationship with the funding agency, they will announce future calls, and your past experience and familiarity with the process helps.

3.19   Acknowledging the Funding Body in the Publications

Due acknowledgment with the details of project ID in the asked format should be done in the publications. Reprints should be made available to the funding body.

3.20   Conclusion

Just as researchers look for funding opportunities to execute the research plans, the funding agencies are also always keen to fund and support well-thought-out ideas. Mastering the art of grant writing requires investing time not only to plan the science behind the research idea but also present it in a skillful manner taking into full consideration the scope and expectations of the funding bodies. The grant applicants should keep abreast of the latest guidelines for the funding program they wish to apply to and should not hesitate to communicate with the funding agency to discuss their ideas even during the initial stages. A transparent communication between the researchers and the funders forms the basis of a fruitful association between the two and is the key to the success of any research funding. Happy writing!

Case Scenario 1
A grant applicant has a researcher friend working in a hospital in the field of tuberculosis. The grant application theme is malaria, and the applicant lists the TB researcher as one of his collaborators, assuming that he could provide samples from the hospital for the proposed study. The application is likely to be rejected by the reviewers due to an inappropriate choice of collaborator.

Case Scenario 2
The applicant demands equal funding for all the years during the study period. However, practically the requirements during each year of the study would be different, and so would the funding demands. Such a proposal is likely to be rejected by the reviewers and flagged as a poorly-thought budget plan.

Case Scenario 3
The applicant approaches the host institution's director and a senior researcher for letters of support from the host institute and as a mentor, respectively. Both of them ask the applicant to prepare a draft of the support letters. The applicant uses the same language and format in both the letters of support and submits along with the application. The reviewers can immediately make out that the letters of support have not been written by the sender.

References

1. Neema S, Chandrashekar L. Research funding-why, when, and how? Indian Dermatol Online J. 2021;12(1):134–8.

2. Kanji S. Turning your research idea into a proposal worth funding. Can J Hosp Pharm. 2015;68 (6):458–64.
3. Formula for Grant Success: CIRM Grant Writing Webinar. https://www.youtube.com/watch?v= A1Zb5I17qGs.
4. Gemayel R, Martin SJ. Writing a successful fellowship or grant application. FEBS J. 2017;284 (22):3771–7.
5. Santen RJ, Barrett EJ, Siragy HM, Farhi LS, Fishbein L, Carey RM. The jewel in the crown: specific aims section of investigator-initiated grant proposals. J Endocr Soc. 2017;1(9): 1194–202.
6. Guyer RA, Schwarze ML, Gosain A, Maggard-Gibbons M, Keswani SG, Goldstein AM. Top ten strategies to enhance grant-writing success. Surgery. 2021;170(6):1727–31.
7. Kan P, Mokin M, Mack WJ, Starke RM, Sheth KN, Albuquerque FC, et al. Strategies for writing a successful National Institutes of Health grant proposal for the early-career neurointerventionalist. J Neurointervent Surg. 2020;13(3):283–6.

Funding Organizations for Science and Health Care

4

Biswajit Dubashi and Balamurugan Ramadass

An investment in knowledge always pays the best interest

Benjamin Franklin

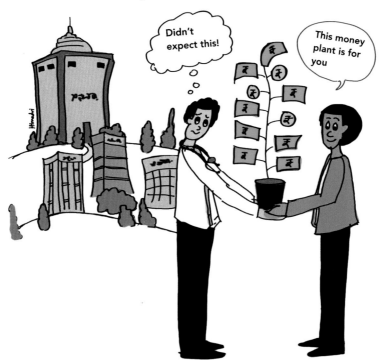

Funding organizations for science and health care

B. Dubashi (✉)
Department of Medical Oncology, Jawaharlal Institute of Postgraduate Medical Education and Research (JIPMER), Pondicherry, India

B. Ramadass
Clinical Biochemistry Laboratory, Department of Biochemistry, Center of Excellence for Clinical Microbiome Research, All India Institute of Medical Sciences (AIIMS) Bhubaneswar, Bhubaneswar, Odisha, India

Objectives
- Recognize various funding organizations globally
- Understand the various areas of focus of the funding organizations

4.1   Introduction

A research project to be successful includes a well-conceptualized idea with a comprehensively written protocol and appropriate execution of the project. The implementation of the project requires funding in terms of manpower, equipment, consumables and drugs, travel expenses for attending workshops, conferences, and institutional administrative charges. Historically, funding for research was small, particularly before the second world war; it was focused on public health concerns, national security, and aeronautical research. Over the years, funding for research across the globe has been steadily increasing. As per a report by UNESCO, the USA spends 2.84% of the GDP and is ranked one, while India spends 0.65% of the GDP and is ranked seventh on research funding. [Ref Research and development expenditure (% of GDP)-India. worldbank.org]. The GERD (Gross Expenditure on R&D) to GDP ratio is a widely used metric which is 0.6–0.8 in India over the last two decades compared to Israel, Japan, USA, China, and the UK, which have a GDP of 4.9, 3.2, 2.7, 2.2, and 1.7, respectively. According to the Organization for Economic Cooperation and Development (OCED), industries carry out 60% of technical, scientific research and development, 20% by universities, and 10% by government institutes. Philanthropists, crowdsourcing, private enterprises, non-profit foundations, and professional associations are among the sources of private research funding. Publication output, citation impact, number of patents, and number of PhDs awarded are all indicators of the outcome. This chapter will describe the importance and types of funding, components of budget-writing, funding opportunities available at national and international levels, and drawbacks of funding.

4.2   How Do Funding Agencies Facilitate or Hinder Research Progress?

Funding organizations can potentially help develop research and education both at basic science and translational levels. The goal is to incentivize research ideas and allocate research funding to deliver scientific progress and eventually economic and social returns. The development of newer drugs and devices requires strengthening basic science research and applying this knowledge for approval in humans. This process is expensive and involves a cost that is not possible by individual funding. Funding organizations can facilitate interdisciplinary research and education by integrating science and technology centers and engineering research centers to partner with industry. As partners (policymakers, clinicians) in creating the proposal, conducting the study, and implementing it, funding agencies support knowledge transfer as an integral component of the research process addressed in the grant proposal. The research funders then disseminate information about funded and completed projects and the implementation of the research in a real-world setting [1].

Funding agencies can influence research conscious or unconscious biases in researchers' work. There is possible favoritism in outcomes of research sponsored by the agency. Biomedical journals have made it imperative to disclose any potential conflicts of interest (COIs). A British study showed that most national and food policy committee members received funding from food companies [2]. A meta-analysis published in 2011 by Cochrane review suggested the possible conflicts of interests [COI] and found they were rarely disclosed. The study reviewed an aggregate of 509 randomized controlled trials, which reported industry as a major funding source (69%). The reported author COI disclosure disclosing industrial, financial ties was seen in 69%. 7% reported funding sources, and none reported the exact author–industry tie-up [3]. In a 2005 study in Nature journal, which surveyed 3247 US researchers who were publicly funded, 15% admitted to changing the design, methodology, or results of their studies due to pressure from the external funding source [4].

4.3 How Do You Get Funding for Research?

Finding funding to do research is significant, and it is exhaustive. More than 10% of an average academician's time is spent on funding and developing research. In India, the success percent of a funding application is about 1 in 10. One way to secure funding for your research is to apply for the grants that best suit you and your team's research experience [5]. The first of the many strategies that can assist a researcher in securing funding opportunities is to convert a research idea into a proposal worth funding. This is a topic for another chapter.

Prelude to funding: a compelling research idea is an essential prelude to developing a research proposal. Before designing your research question, spend as much time as necessary for a thorough literature review. Perform essential scoping exercises to confirm that the research question is novel and hasn't been answered. Most importantly, it should be relevant to the country and others in the field of interest.

Where is the money? Finding a suitable source of funding opportunities is sometimes the most challenging part of applying for funding. Apply to one of the many government funding opportunities available may come with specific eligibility criteria. Primarily, researchers may have to be affiliated with an eligible institution or organization recognized under the state or central govt. or institute of national repute for academic standing. Many institute of national importance offers institutional level opportunities for research funding to generate essential proof of concept. In India, every researcher knows the major funding agency, like the ICMR, DBT, DST, and CSIR. Still, there are many others like charities and non-government organizations that are offering more than ever before. For example, private or charitable foundations [e.g., Sree Padmavathi Foundation

(SreePVF) has called for Sree Ramakrishna Paramahamsa Research Grant 2021, offering up to 3 crores for cutting-edge research proposals]. Particularly, in this chapter, various funding options nationally and internationally are enumerated for ready reference. As a service to the researchers, the institute research administration should provide necessary details on sources for funding for research and other scholarly activities.

Look everywhere; sometimes, looking at standard options within the country may not be sufficient. Most research is collaborative and happens internationally; therefore, better options would be to look for funds worldwide. If you google "research funding options" or "funding search tools," most will get over a thousand results. Most of them will be articles describing how to secure funding, such as this chapter. Others are usually university funding search options, government portals, or paid search portals that may require subscription by an individual or by the institute. Research administration in top-ranking universities provides information on funding sources to their researchers. Primarily, research offices in these universities enlist top funding search tools that they recommend and or subscribe to. One of the most commonly subscribed funding search tools is PIVOT. This database is accessible only by email-IDs of membership subscriptions by the universities for their faculty and staff. PIVOT is a comprehensive editorially curated science funding opportunity database that keeps over 400,000 global funding options. It provides information on grants, fellowships, social sciences, community outreach programs, and other funding information from government, corporate, domestic and international sources. PIVOT automatically matches scholar profiles via its funding advisor recommendation engine, provides discoverability of potential collaborators, provides tailored funding recommendations, and provides insights from previously awarded grants. Elsevier hosts the funding institutional platform, which is equivalent to PIVOT. Funding institutional platform lists over 15,000 ongoing calls for proposals for funding opportunities with details of over three million research grants awarded from a wide range of government and private funders worldwide. However, the equivalent of these funding search sites specifically for various countries is not available.

Targeted search: PIVOT or funding institutional platform can be tempting to fish on wider waters. Realistically, these approaches are meant for deep-water fishing. This essentially means enhancing focus and effort on opportunities that are best suited for success. For example, there is no benefit in applying for a Center of Excellence grant or a core grant by an early-stage researcher. Another typical example could be that some grants are specifically targeted at women, minorities, or people from LMI countries. Utilizing such targeted options can improve your success chances. For a targeted search, the crucial prerequisite is that you are an active researcher and looking for opportunities constantly for your next or follow-through idea.

Provide Potential; Global funding opportunities are available based on three imperative components: idea, insight, and collaboration. The community of science maintains a database of researcher profiles and their expertise. This can help connect geographically and institutionally to identify potential collaborators according to their skill set. On the other hand, such databases will also expose researchers who don't have long publication history or a high citation index. Also, other metrics that focus on academics and other features like online attention of the research, collaborative network, news, and social media are built in to encourage an early-career researcher who otherwise may fall victim to a traditional database. However, a good proportion of researchers get activated only when they encounter a "call for proposal." These researchers approach any "Call for Proposals" without 5Ps, Preliminary experience, Published data, Prior funding history, Proper collaborative effort, Partially developed the idea, and most importantly, a passively prepared proposal. These are typically signs of inconsistent researchers and or novices. They have to find a suitable guide to coach themselves on how they can apply for successful funding.

4.4 What are the Types of Research Funding?

Research fundings are usually four types namely formula, continuation funding, competitive funding and pass through funding. Competitive funding is based on the evaluation of a reviewer or team of reviewers on the merits of the application. Formula funding is provided to predetermined recipients who are usually allocated to eligible entities depending on the consensus criteria meeting the minimum requirements of the application. Continuation funding is a program that offers extension grants for current ongoing projects. Pass-through funding is provided to an organization that then sub-distributes the fund for research activity either as a competitive or non-competitive process.

Funding research usually comes from three sources, namely Corporations (research and development departments) and Government (universities and specialized government agencies like research councils and NGOs dedicated to developing a cure for various diseases like tuberculosis, AIDS, malaria, and cancer [6].

The areas covered for research funding are broad and include open funding for core areas of research like communicable and non-communicable diseases with themes that may change from time to time depending on the research priority. Fundings are available for individual and collaborative projects as part of the extramural ad hoc proposals. The postgraduates and PhD students can avail of funding for the thesis to attend conferences for paper presentations and workshops. There is funding available for young women scientists and junior and senior-level faculty. There are grants available for developing centers for advanced research like pharmacogenomics, molecular genetics, clinical trials, etc. There is separate funding available for Medical Innovations. International Collaborative fundings with the governmental agency of India and other countries like the Indo-Swiss, Indo-French, Indo-UK, and Indo-US are available, which requires identification of collaborating institutes and shared funding from both the countries.

4.5   Information Regarding Various Funding Agencies (National and International Agencies)

4.5.1   Status of Research Funding in India

The Gross Expenditure on R&D (GERD) from 2017—was primarily initiated by the govt. sector, wherein the central govt. spent 45.4% while the business enterprises, state governments, higher education, and public sector industry spent 36.8%, 6.4%, 6.8%, and 4.6%, respectively. Among the central government GERD, 93% of the GERD contribution was incurred by 12 major scientific agencies. According to the Research and Development Statistics that were published by the Department of Science and Technology, Ministry of Science and Technology, Government of India in the year 2019–2020, the Defence Research and Development Organisation (DRDO) accounts for the major share (31.6%) of Gross Expenditure on R&D. Based on the type of research done nationally the percentage share of expenditure of applied research, experimental development, basic research, and other activities are 36.9%, 32.4%, 23.9%, and 6.8%, respectively.

The details of the national and international funding agencies, including the thrust areas of research, available grants, and nature of support, are described [6–9].

S. no.	Name of the agency	Website	Remarks
National agency			
1.	Defence Research and Development Organisation	https://www.drdo.gov.in/	
2.	Department of Science and Technology (DST)	http://www.dst.gov.in/	
3.	SERB (Science and Engineering Research Board)	http://www.serb.gov.in/home.php	
4.	Department of Biotechnology (DBT)	http://www.dbtindia.nic.in/	
5.	Indian Council of Medical Research (ICMR)	http://www.icmr.nic.in/	
6.	Council of Scientific and Industrial Research (CSIR)	http://www.csir.res.in/	
7.	AYUSH	https://main.ayush.gov.in/	Department of Ayurveda, Yoga and Naturopathy, Unani, Siddha, and Homeopathy
8.	UGC Faculty Research Promotion Scheme (UGC-FRPS)	http://ugcfrps.ac.in/uohyd/	Mid-Career Awards, Start-Up Grants, and fellowships for basic science research
9.	Board of Research and Nuclear Science (BRNS)	http://www.barc.gov.in/brns/index.htm	

(continued)

S. no.	Name of the agency	Website	Remarks
10.	Newton-Bhabha Fund (British Council)	http://www.newtonfund.ac.uk/about/about-partnering-countries/India	
11.	AD (Indo-German)	http://www.daaddelhi.org/en/14498/index.html	
12.	Indo-French Centre for the Promotion of Advanced Research (IFCPAR)	http://www.cefipra.org/	
13.	Department of Atomic Energy (DAE)	http://dae.nic.in	
14.	Tata Institute of Fundamental Research (TIFR)	http://www.tifr.res.in/	
15.	All India Council for Technical Education (AICTE)	http://www.aicte-india.org/	Schemes promoting research and institutional development
16.	Indian National Science Academy	https://www.insaindia.res.in/	Promote scientific knowledge in India and its practical application to national welfare concerns, as well as coordination between scientific academies, groups, institutes, and government scientific departments and services. The scientists can work in an R&D center, university, or institution in India for a period of 3 years in their chosen field
16.	National Cancer Grid	https://tmc.gov.in/ncg/	A network of major cancer centers, research institutes, patient groups, and charitable organizations across India with the mission of establishing uniform patient care standards for cancer prevention, diagnosis, and treatment, providing specialized training and education in oncology and facilitating collaborative basic, translational, and clinical cancer research Multicentric cancer research projects
International agency			
1.	National Institutes of Health (NIH)	https://www.nih.gov/	The National Institutes of Health (NIH) conducts research

(continued)

S. no.	Name of the agency	Website	Remarks
			in all areas of health, with the majority of its work being extramural. The funding mechanism, properly speaking, takes an untargeted approach and hence does not strictly prioritize a single area of research
2.	European Commissions	https://ec.europa.eu/info/index_en	The EC has two sub-programs that involve health-related research, that is, FP7—Cooperation program—Health theme/Health Directorate and European Research Council (ERC) since it is not limited to just health-related research
3.	UK Medical Research Council (MRC)	https://mrc.ukri.org/	Medical professionals from the UK and across the globe are encouraged by the MRC to accept intramural and extramural research
4.	Institut National De La Santé et De La Recherché Médicale (INSERM)	https://www.inserm.fr/en/home/	A purely intramural public funding institute that focuses on French medical research
5.	Wellcome Trust	https://wellcome.org/	A philanthropic organization that primarily invests in extramural research situated in the Great Britain Republic
6.	Canadian Institutes of Health Research (CIHR)	https://cihr-irsc.gc.ca/e/193.html	Based in Canada, involves purely extramural research and targeted and untargeted research
7.	Australian National Health and Medical Research Council (NHMRC)	https://www.nhmrc.gov.au/	Untargeted research is a major priority, and it relies on extramural researchers
8.	Howard Hughes Medical Institute (HHMI)	https://www.hhmi.org/	A philanthropic organization in the USA, extramural and untargeted
9.	Deutsche Forschungsgemeinschaft/German Research Foundation (GFR)	https://www.research-in-germany.org/en/research-funding	A German Institute, extramural both targeted and targeted research

(Adapted from the respective official websites)

4.5.1.1 Department of Science and Technology (DST)

The DST formulates policies related to science and technology, matters related to the scientific advisory committee to the cabinet, promoting of new areas of technology, and provides grants in aid to research institutions and scientific associations. The area of funding includes scientific and engineering research, technology development, and women scientist programs [6–9].

S. no.	Name of the program	Description
Science and technology		
	Mega facilities for basic research	To create mega science facilities and launch mega science projects in and out of the country
	"Innovation in Science Pursuit for Inspired Research (INSPIRE) programme"	Develop creative pursuit of science and attract talent to the study of science at an early stage. INSPIRE Scheme has included three programs and five components. They are "(a) Scheme for Early Attraction of Talents for Science (SEATS), (b) Scholarship for Higher Education (SHE), and (c) Assured Opportunity for Research Careers (AORC). The five components include INSPIRE awards_MANAK, INSPIRE Internship, INSPIRE Scholarship, INSPIRE Fellowship, INSPIRE Faculty"
	R&D Infrastructure (FIST, SAIFs, PURSE, SATHI)	Provide funds for the improvement of infrastructure in universities and institutes, "Sophisticated Analytical Instrument Facilities (SAIFs), Promotion of University Research and Scientific Excellence (PURSE), and Sophisticated Analytical and Technical Help Institutes (SATHI)"
	Science and Technology of Yoga and Meditation (SATYAM)	Basic themes being covered under SATYAM include (1) investigations into the effects of yoga and meditation on physical and mental health and well-being and (2) investigations into the basic processes and mechanisms of yoga and meditation on the body, brain, and mind
	Program for Science Students	Kishore Vaigyanik Protsahan Yojana (KVPY)—to identify students with talent and aptitude for research. National Science Olympiad Program covering Mathematics and Sciences, including Astronomy
	Swarnajayanti Fellowships	A selected number of young scientists with a proven track record are provided special assistance and support to enable them to pursue basic research
	National Science and Technology Management Information System (NSTMIS)	Collection, collation, analysis, and dissemination of information on resources devoted to S&T activities in the country
	Science and Engineering Research Board (SERB)	Described separately below
	Cognitive Science Research Initiative (CSRI)	A platform for the scientific community to work for better solutions to challenges

(continued)

S. no.	Name of the program	Description
		related to cognitive disorders and social issues through various psychological tools and batteries, early diagnosis and better therapies, intervention technologies, and rehabilitation programs. Individual R&D projects, multicentric mega projects, post-doctoral fellowship, support for schools, training, workshops, conferences
	VAJRA (Visiting Advanced Joint Research) Faculty Scheme	The Indian collaborator and the overseas faculty will jointly frame a research plan, and the application duly endorsed by the Head of the Institution will be submitted online by the Indian collaborator. The residency period of the VAJRA Faculty in India would be for a minimum of 1 month and a maximum of 3 months a year
Technology development		
	Technical Research Centres Programme	Technical Research Centres (TRCs) were established during FY 2015–2016 in the following DST institutions: Sree Chitra Tirunal Institute for Medical Sciences and Technology (SCTIMST), Trivandrum, International Advanced Research Centre for Powder Metallurgy and New Materials (ARCI), Hyderabad, Jawaharlal Nehru Centre for Advanced Scientific Research (JNCASR), Bengaluru, Indian Association for the Cultivation of Science (IACS), Kolkata, S.N. Bose National Centre for Basic Sciences, Kolkata. Research development, industry–institute partnership programs. The specific research programs are available on the website
	Technology Development and Transfer	Technology development projects include materials, devices, and processes **Core Areas for inviting proposals under TDP** Advanced Manufacturing Technologies (AMT) Waste Management Technologies (WMT) Biomedical Device and Technology Development Programme (BDTD) Device Development Programme (DDP) Technology Development Programme (TDP) DHI-DST Technology Platform for Electric Mobility (TPEM) Science and Heritage Research Initiative (SHRI)

(continued)

S. no.	Name of the program	Description
	Patent Facilitation Programme (PFP)	Provide Patent information as a vital input to R&D, Patent/IPR facilitation to academic Institutions and Government R&D Institutions, IPR policy input to government, and conducting training and awareness programs on IPR in the country
	National Council for Science and Technology Communication (NCSTC)	Communicate Science and Technology to the masses stimulate scientific and technological temper and coordinate and orchestrate such efforts throughout the country through the National Award for Science and Technology Communication 2021 communicating science using folk media; use of mass and digital media for science communication and popularization; use of social media in science and technology popularization
International collaboration		
	"Indo-French Centre for Promotion of Advanced Research (IFCPAR/CEFIPRA), Indo-US Science and Technology Forum (IUSSTF) Indo-German Science and Technology Centre (IGSTC)"	The IC Division currently supports three binational S&T Centers, which are independent entities established under inter-governmental arrangements with France, the USA, and Germany
Women Scientist program		
	Gender Advancement for Transforming Institutions (GATI)	Gender Advancement in Research at the institutional level
	Women Scientist Scheme (A–C)	WOS A (Women Scientist Scheme A) supports research in basic and applied sciences. WOS B (Women Scientist Scheme B) encourages S and T interventions that benefit society. Women Scientist Scheme C (WOS C) intends to train women for a year in order to create a pool of women scientists in order to generate and manage intellectual property rights in India

4.5.1.2 SERB (Science and Engineering Research Board)

SERB is a statutory body established through the act of parliament. The board has the financial and administrative powers to decide on research areas. SERB supports research in frontier areas of science and engineering. The common grants include the Core Research Grant scheme for scientists and the start-up research grant as a one-time career grant to assist scientists in initiating research careers in institutions. They have a special program for women scientists (SERB women excellence), a one-time award for women below 40 years. They have a special program for young scientists less than 35 years of age to conduct independent research. The

Intensification of Research in High priority Areas (IRHPA) program is supported by SERB. The board also offers JC Bose National fellowship to scientists for outstanding performance and contribution to science. The Ramanujam fellowship is provided to scientists and engineers from all over the world to take up scientific research positions in India. They also provide financial support on a competitive basis for organizing scientific events. The Scientific and Useful Profound Research Advancement (SUPRA) is a scheme for high-quality proposals. The empowerment and equity opportunities for excellence in science is a grant for a post-doctoral PhD belonging to SC/ST caste [6–9].

4.5.1.3 Department of Biotechnology (DBT)

The Department of Biotechnology (DBT), Ministry of Science and Technology, Government of India has the mandate of promoting and nurturing biotechnology in the country. The thrust areas of funding include the promotion of large-scale use of biotechnology, support of research and development and manufacturing in biology, promoting university and industry interaction, and setting up centers of excellence [6–9].

S. no.	Name of the program	Remarks
Medical Biotechnology		
	Vaccine research and development	Key initiatives to support basic and translational research for strengthening vaccine science that is currently under implementation include the (1) Indo-US Vaccine Action Programme (VAP), (2) National Biopharma Mission (NBM), (3) Ind-CEPI Mission, and (4) Mission COVID Suraksha
	Public Health and Nutrition	The program was initiated in 1994 as "Food and Nutrition." The thrust from the beginning of the program was to develop technological and clinical solutions for nutrition-related problems like malnutrition, anemia, diarrhea, stunting, etc.
	Stem cells and regenerative medicine	To promote basic, early, and late translational research in the area of stem cell and regenerative medicine and to promote scientific interactions and collaborations among clinicians and researchers, building capacity in this area
	Biomedical Engineering and Biodesign	The objective of biomedical engineering is to foster and support innovative ideas in the fields of biomaterials for various therapeutic/biomedical applications; biomedical devices, implants and bioinstrumentation; biomedical sensors; bio-imaging for improved diagnostics/existing medical equipment; tissue engineering and other allied areas for the development of affordable healthcare products. **The overall focus of bio-design is on the invention and early-stage development of affordable implants and devices for the country**
	Infectious disease biology	Identifying novel pathogens by deciphering the molecular structure and functions of existing viral,

(continued)

S. no.	Name of the program	Remarks
		bacterial, fungal, and parasitic diseases
		Extending knowledge of infection processes, pathogenicity, virulence, host–pathogen interactions, drug-resistance development in illnesses like tuberculosis, therapeutic repurposing for infectious disorders, and antimicrobial resistance
		Development of indigenous diagnostic platforms and technologies that are dependable
		Identifying possible targets for the development of innovative broad-spectrum therapeutic techniques, repurposing of drugs for infectious diseases, and antimicrobial resistance
		Development of indigenous diagnostic platforms and technologies that are dependable
		Determining prospective targets for creating fresh broad-spectrum therapeutic techniques
	Chronic/Life disease-Cancer, Diabetes and other biology	Focus areas include
		1. Noninvasive cancer diagnostics
		2. Cancer immunology and cancer immunotherapy and clinical trials
		3. Diabetes and its complications
		4. Respiratory diseases
		5. Cardiovascular diseases
		6. Bone biology and osteoporosis
		7. Lifestyle and chronic diseases
		8. National Alliance for Translational Research in Autoimmune Diseases
		9. Autism and behavioral disorders in children
		10. Acute encephalopathy/encephalitis syndrome
	Human Genetics and Genome Analysis	**Priority areas**
		1. Precision health
		2. Rare genetic disorders
		3. Mutation spectrum of genetic and complex diseases in the Indian population
		4. Genetic epidemiology of multifactorial lifestyle diseases
		5. Translational research
	New Drug Development and biogenerics	
Building capacity		
	Teaching and training	Postgraduates, PhD, post-doctoral fellowships, research in universities, national and international fellowship, awards, popularization and promotion of biotechnology and building critical mass of science leaders
		The common and popular fellowships offered include DBT Junior Research, DBT Research Associateship program, and Ramalingaswami Re-entry fellowship
		DBT-Wellcome Trust—aims to improve the biomedical research landscape in India through mechanisms fellowship supports exceptional

(continued)

S. no.	Name of the program	Remarks
		researchers at Indian institutions and facilitates the recruitment of highly trained and qualified scientists from overseas. This is done through fellowship program with three types of fellowships early, intermediate, and senior fellowships
	International Co-operation	
	Bilateral, Multilateral, and other Partnerships	Focus and promote collaborative research to solve a myriad of socio-economic as well as environmental challenges. Countries in Europe (the UK, Finland, Denmark, Switzerland, Sweden, Brazil, South Korea, Cuba, Australia, Canada, and many other countries)
	Promoting Biotechnology in North-East region	Research and Development Biotech research facilities Capacity building programs
	Mission programs	1. Atal Jai Anusandhan Biotech UNaTI GARBH-Ini, Mission Antimicrobial Resistance (AMR), Ind-CEPI MISSION, Mission Innovation: Accelerating the Clean, Energy Innovation 2. Development of Biofortified and Protein-rich wheat: contributing to POSHANAbhiyan 3. National Biopharma Mission 4. Phytopharmaceutical Mission 5. Biotech-Krishi Innovation Science 6. Application Network (Biotech-KISAN) 7. DBT-Unique Methods of Management of inherited Disorders (UMMID) initiative 8. Genome India 9. Mission Programme on Characterization of Genetic Resources
	Translational and industrial developmental programs	Development of Biotech parks and Incubators, Make in India and Startup India program, patent facilitation
	Special programs	Biotechnology for societal development BioCare program for career development

4.5.1.4 Indian Council of Medical Research (ICMR)

ICMR is the pinnacle in India with respect to the formulation, coordination, and promotion of biomedical research. Control and management of communicable diseases, fertility control, maternity and child health, nutritional disorders control, development of alternative healthcare delivery schemes, containment of environmental and occupational health problems within safe limits, and non-communicable diseases such as cancer, diabetes, and cardiovascular diseases are all common research priorities [6–9].

ICMR-DHR Programs		
1.	SHARP (Support for Human resources Academics and Research Programmes)	Long-term fellowships for young Indian biomedical scientists, short-term fellowships for senior Indian biomedical scientists,

(continued)

ICMR-DHR Programs

		fellowships for scientists from developing countries, NRI and OCI Nurturing Clinical Scientists Scheme, short-term studentship for MBBS/BDS students, MD/MS/PhD fellowship, student fellowships (JRF, SRF, Research Associates, post-doctoral fellowship, long-term and short-term fellowships in India, biomedical research career program, schemes for senior scientist ICMR-Emeritus Scientists, financial support for travel/thesis/workshops
2.	Extramural Research Program (ad hoc)	Types of Extramural Research Program include short duration, low-cost proposals, ad hoc project—Investigator defined, Task Force project—Solve a predefined problem (Centrally identified), Cohort study, National Registry, Centers of Advanced Research (CAR), Capacity building/support for sustained high-quality research
3.	Adjunct Faculty Scheme	This will enable NRI/PIO and foreign nationals with strong Indian collaboration from the overseas scientific community to participate and contribute to biomedical research in India. The adjunct faculty will undertake research in the field of biomedical Research and ICMR priority areas
4.	Medical innovation fund	To support the testing and validation of unique and highly creative ideas, even if they have a significant risk of failure, in order to expedite medical innovation. This scheme is open to only the council's scientists for support
5.	International travel by non-ICMR faculty	Provide financial assistance for presenting a research paper or chairing a session as also delivering a lecture/delivering a keynote address in an international scientific event to non-ICMR biomedical scientists
6.	ICMR chairs—Dr. C.G. Pandit national chairs, Dr. A.S. Paintal Distinguished Scientist Chairs	ICMR Chairs should work preferably at ICMR Hqrs./Institutes. With the remuneration of Rs. 2.00 lakh per month

4.5.1.5 Council of Scientific and Industrial Research (CSIR)

The Council of Scientific and Industrial Research is an autonomous body for its excellence in R&D and S&T innovations. With a network of 38 national laboratories, 39 outreach centers, one innovation complex, and three units, CSIR has a presence all over India [10, 11].

S. no.	Name of the program	Remarks
	Funding of Extra Mural Research Schemes to promote R&D	Healthcare (HTC) Facility Creation Projects (FCP) aim at building new infrastructure or upgrading the existing one to meet new technological challenges and to generate revenues at the CSIR laboratories
	CSIR Technology Awards	Life sciences
	Junior Research Fellowship (NET)	Junior Research Fellowship and lectureship and CSIR to be supported by UGC
	Shyama Prasad Mukherji Fellowship (SPMF)	To identify and nurture budding scientific talent in pursuit of scientific research
	Senior Research Fellowship (SRF) and Research Associateship (RA)	
	Junior Research Fellowship for GATE qualified pharmacy graduates (JRF-GATE)	
	Bilateral International Projects	Scientific Interactions through Exchange Visits
	Travel/Conference Grants	

4.5.1.6 Ayush

Ayush was formed to revive the comprehensive knowledge of traditional Indian medical systems by raising educational standards for Indian medical systems, strengthening existing research institutions, and ensuring time-bound research programs on ailments for which these systems offer effective treatments [7].

S. no.	Name of the program	Remarks
1.	• Central Sector Scheme	**AYURSWASTHYA YOJANA**—Main components include public health, sports medicine, and upgradation of facilities to the Center of Excellence **AYURGYAN Scheme**—Capacity Building and Continued Medical Education, Research and Innovation in Ayush (Erstwhile Extra Mural Research Scheme)
2.	• Centrally Sponsored Schemes	NATIONAL AYUSH MISSION (NAM)—(a) To provide cost-effective and equitable AYUSH health care throughout the country by improving access to the services. (b) To revitalize and strengthen the AYUSH systems making them prominent medical streams in addressing the health care of the society. (c) To improve educational institutions capable of imparting quality AYUSH education. (d) To promote the adoption of quality standards of AYUSH drugs and make available the sustained supply of AYUSH raw materials
3.	• Financial Sanctions	Quality control of Ayush drugs, development of Ayush industry cluster, upgradation of the center of excellence

(continued)

S. no.	Name of the program	Remarks
4.	• Award Scheme of CCRUM	Best Research Paper Award, Young Scientist Award, Life-Time Achievement Award, Best Teacher Award
5.	• AYUSH Centre of Excellence (ACE) Programme	(1) Centre of Excellence in AYUSH Research, (2) Centre of Excellence in AYUSH Health Services, (3) Centre of Excellence in AYUSH multispecialty services, (4) Centre of Excellence in AYUSH Pharmacology/Pharmacognosy, (5) Centre of Excellence in AYUSH Pharmaceutics, (6) Centre of Excellence in Ayurveda Biology, (7) Centre of Excellence in Medicinal Plants

4.6   How to Write a Budget Proposal?

By definition, a budget is a detailed statement of estimated expenses to support a funded project. An effective estimate of the proposed project should be within the budget limits prescribed by the funding agency, and it should be backed up by a clear justification to assist the reviewers in determining how the project will be conducted.

Typically, a budget consists of

Direct costs:

1. Non-Recurring Costs: Depending on a project, there may be requirements that are expected to happen one time at the beginning of the study and not routinely. For example, equipment that is not available in the institute, or there may be the need for a vehicle for public health project proposals. These are one-time expenses and are non-recurring in nature.
2. Personnel cost: For example, Scientist, Assistant Professor, Post-doctoral Fellow, Medical Officers, Senior Research Fellow, Junior Research Fellow, Research Assistant, Laboratory Managers, Technicians, Project Co-ordinators, Social Workers, Dietitian, Fieldworker, Attenders, or ASHA workers.
3. Materials and supply: It is a broad category that includes all non-capital items like computers and electronic equipment as well as laboratory consumables. These are expenses that occur at regular intervals and are recurring in nature.
4. Travel: Travel costs are usually for expenses that include transport costs for field visits or for expenses project employees incur during travel to study sites. Also, travel costs include transportation, lodging, and living costs incurred by PI or project Fellows for official project-related trips. It may also include trips to present research data to the funding agency or to conferences nationally or internationally.
5. Contingency: This head is typically for all the "catch-all" expenses. The funds in this can be utilized for any expenses that are not defined under any of the above heads and are unexpected in nature. Most importantly, it is a backup fund for unforeseen expenses.

Indirect costs:

This can be simply called the overhead charges.

Usually, indirect costs are a fixed percentage of the direct costs. These percentages again vary with the principal investigator's institute. Overhead charges are utilized differently based on the institute policies. However, it is broadly for the institute to support the funded proposal.

Budget Justification: A well-planned budget is accompanied by a suitable explanation. A realistic budget is only complete with appropriate justification for the expenses conceived. A good budget justification allows the reviewer or the sponsor to envision the principal investigator's clarity and may provide more evidence to support the application. Funding agencies usually rely on reviewers to approve the budget. A good budget justification may support the reviewer and the funding agency to not reduce or discard budget categories.

4.7 Evaluation Process and Measurement of Efficiency for Research Funding

4.7.1 Evaluation Process

The funding agencies have a detailed evaluation process before sanctioning the grant. The application is examined internally by the initial screening committee for completeness, objectives of the project, status of technology, competence of the applicant, and budget. Preliminary discussions with the applicant and the technology supplier, as well as a request for the candidate to give a presentation, may also be part of the screening process. If an application is not meeting the criteria for financial assistance and would fit under another scheme accordingly, the applicants are advised to revise. The protocols are then sent for external review to experts in the field. The experts review the novelty of the project, soundness of the methodology, outcomes, the applicant's potential to complete the project, budget, and feasibility. A score is provided, which is reviewed by the funding agency [12].

Most funding agencies have a Project Evaluation Committee (PEC) which finally recommends the project for funding.

The PEC evaluates the application for its scientific, technological, commercial, and financial merits. The evaluation criteria shall include:

1. Scientific novelty, quality, and feasibility
2. Prospects for broad application and the benefits expected to emanate from commercialization
3. Sufficiency of the effort proposed
4. The capacity of the R&D institution(s) in the suggested action network
5. Enterprise's organizational and commercial competence as well as the internal accruals
6. Substantiality of the budget pattern submitted
7. Objectives, endpoints, and milestones that are quantifiable
8. Credentials of the entrepreneur

4.7.2 Monitoring and Efficiency of Funding

Group monitoring workshops keep track of the authorized projects' progress. This is particularly beneficial to the project's success because it allows for mid-course modifications and the recommendation of initiatives for support. While approving the grant, the review of progress in the annual group monitoring workshop/field visit is also taken into account. Given the reality on the ground, there is substantial flexibility in terms of finance as well as amending or abandoning authorized project objectives. Publication output, citation impact, number of patents, and number of PhDs awarded are all indicators of the outcome. The impact assessment is based on the acceptability of the intervention, techno-economic viability, and potential replicability.

4.8 Conclusion

A successful project requires a well-written balanced funding to make the research outcome a success. There are numerous international and national, private as well as governmental organizations that provide funding for various medical research which includes basic science (human and animal research), observational, interventional, and public health research. An understanding of the different goals and objectives of the funding agencies and keeping track of calls for proposals are important for a successful outcome of funding.

Case Scenario 1

Mr. X, Principal investigator from Chennai, wants to write a project on "How the molecular and pharmacogenetic markers in relation to clinical response and toxicity to drugs in children with blood cancer possibly different in India compared to other countries?" He needs to collaborate with an international researcher and needs to apply for funds for the project.

1. Name two international funding agencies which may be suitable for funding?
2. What are the guidelines for the transfer of biological materials out of the country?

Case Scenario 2

Ms. C is a lead investigator in Oncology and has applied for funding for a multicenter project on a clinical drug trial involving ten centers. The study is a randomized control trial and involves data collection, biological samples, administration of an investigational drug, and monitoring of toxicity. She also needs to take professional indemnity insurance.

Discuss the various heads under which she needs to prepare the budget to successfully complete the project.

References

1. Tetroe JM, Graham ID, Foy R, et al. Health research funding agencies' support and promotion of knowledge translation: an international study. Milbank Q. 2008;86(1):125–55. https://doi.org/10.1111/j.1468-0009.2007.00515.x.
2. Nestle M. Food company sponsorship of nutrition research and professional activities: a conflict of interest? Public Health Nutr. 2001;4(5):1015–22. https://doi.org/10.1079/phn2001253.
3. Cochrane Collaboration. How well do meta-analyses disclose conflicts of interests in underlying research studies. Amsterdam: Elsevier; 2011.
4. Martinson BC, Anderson MS, de Vries R. Scientists behaving badly. Nature. 2005;435(7043): 737–8. https://doi.org/10.1038/435737a.
5. Srinivasan K, Fredrick J, Gupta R, Singh N. Funding opportunities for health research in India—a technical scan. Indian J Public Health. 2020;64:421–7.
6. Gondaliya AV, Shah KV. Funding agencies in India for research in science and technology. Pharma Sci Monit. 2013;4:252–73.
7. https://www.healthresearchfunders.org/health-research-funding-organizations/.
8. https://www.fic.nih.gov/Funding/NonNIH.
9. https://www.nitt.edu/home/icsr/funding_agencies.pdf.
10. https://conductscience.com/top-10-health-funding-organizations/.
11. https://www.aicte-india.org/opportunities/students/research-funds.
12. Sandström U, Van den Besselaar P. Funding, evaluation, and the performance of national research systems. J Informet. 2018;12:365–84.

Vigneshvar Chandrasekaran

> *Surround yourself with only people who are going to lift you higher*
>
> *Oprah Winfrey*

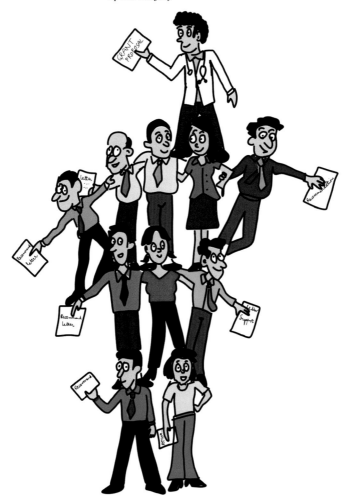

Obtaining letters of support

© The Author(s), under exclusive license to Springer Nature Singapore Pte Ltd. 2023
S. C. Parija, V. Kate (eds.), *Grant writing for medical and healthcare professionals*,
https://doi.org/10.1007/978-981-19-7018-4_5

Objectives
- Understand the concept of Letters of Support
- List the possible providers of Letters of Support
- How to apply for a Letter of Support
- Delineate various components of a Letter of Support
- Appreciate the impact of Letters of Support in the grant application

5.1 Introduction

A research having a significant impact in any field by its virtue involves various components such as research materials, the equipment, and the research personnel [1]. The costs involved in the above-mentioned processes make research grants an essential and most sought-after aspect among researchers of almost all disciplines. The funding through grants can influence the growth and productivity of the concerned field [2]. Further, the progress of a researcher in the academic echelon is frequently assessed based on the quantity and quality of the funds received [3]. Hence, writing for grants becomes a requisite skill for any avid researcher [4].

A research grant proposal which is concise and readily understandable can have higher chances for acceptance by the funding agencies [1]. However, the writeup for the grant is only a part among many in a research proposal. Among such vital components, Letters of Support have a prominent place in application for grants. Letters of Support are a requisite in grant applications for many major funding agencies, both national and global.

5.2 Letters of Support—What are They?

Letters of Support are essentially recommendations or testimonials by an external agency of merit towards the grant proposal [5]. In essence, a Letter of Support is a statement of credibility provided to the grant applicant by other reputable individuals or organizations. Further, the letter of support can also act as a medium explaining the role of the contributors in the project and their expertise [1].

The Letters of Support can act as an assurance for the reviewers of the funding agencies about the direction of the grant proposal [6]. The presence of a letter of support implies that the providers of the letter are confident of the delivery of the proposed results [7]. Letters of Support are usually expected where there is a collaboration of multiple stakeholders or agencies in the project [8]. Letters of Support can be a gamechanger in the current scenario, where there is an increased competition for grants amid a reduced budgets for grants [3].

V. Chandrasekaran (✉)
Department of Psychiatry, Mahatma Gandhi Medical College and Research Institute, Sri Balaji Vidyapeeth, Pondicherry, India

5.3   Who can Provide a Letter of Support?

The sources for obtaining a letter of support include
- Stakeholders/collaborators in the research project. For example, patient recruitment team, laboratory team, etc.
- Individuals or agencies who will be beneficiaries of the research project. For example, the pharmaceutical company providing the medications for the trial.
- Another funding agency/non-profit organizations/non-governmental organizations. For example, charitable institutions, private non-profit foundations, etc.

5.4   Applying for a Letter of Support

5.4.1   Identify the Providers of the Letters

The initial step before applying for Letters of Support would be to identify the individuals or organizations who might be stakeholders in the current research project (Fig. 5.1).

5.4.2   Meeting with the Providers of the Letters

A meeting with such stakeholders with a presentation of the project in detail including the objectives, the methodology, and the expected outcomes can go a long way in procuring a letter of support. Further, an emphasis on the benefits for the

Fig. 5.1 The stepwise process of acquiring a Letter of Support

Identifying the potential providers of Letters of Support based on the research proposal

Meeting with such providers and presentation of the proposal

Requisition for the letter of support based on the format given by the funding agency

Attaching the Letters of Support in the grant application

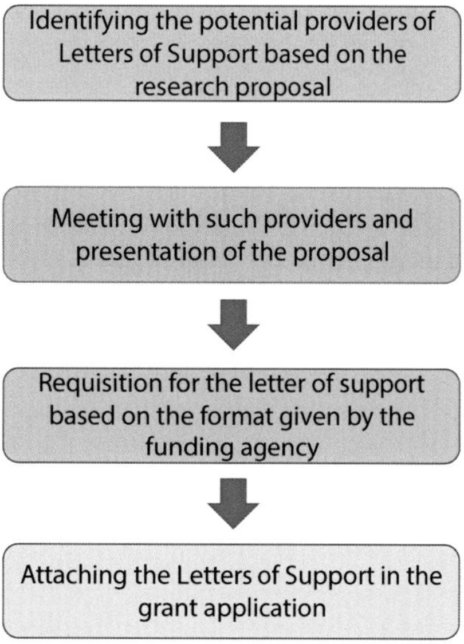

stakeholder with respect to the project can result in a positive response for the request to provide a letter of support.

5.4.3   Requisition for the Letter of Support

After the presentation, a formal mail to the stakeholders requesting for the letter of support must be made without much delay after the day of presentation. The mail should preferably enclose the concept proposal and the fund application.

In certain instances, the funding agencies may require the letter of support in a particular format or template which can be forwarded to the providers of the Letter of Support. A letter of support in line with the expectations of the funding agency will be preferred over other formats.

5.5   Components of a Letter of Support

A Letter of Support should contain the following components [6, 8]
- **Opening statement:** A statement about the research project and the fund application.
- **Middle part:** A brief explanation about the relationship between the fund applicant and the individual/organization providing the Letter of Support. Any collaborations between the supporting party and the fund applicant, if any, a brief mention about the same rather than a formal agreement or Memorandum of Understanding (MoU) is to be included.
- **Closing statement/Conclusion:** The provider of the Letter of Support expresses an explicit statement supporting the research project and the researcher's application for funds. This statement serves as a mention of the commitment of the provider of the support letter towards the project.

It is implied that a Letter of Support should include the credentials of the supporting individual/organization, preferably in the official letter head with signature and seal [7].

The Letters of Support from various stakeholders can be combined or presented individually in the appropriate sections as outlined by the funding agency in its application instructions [9].

The Letters of Support should be relevant and appropriate to the research project for which the grant is being sought. The quality of the letters plays a more decisive role in awarding the grant than the number of letters [6].

5.6   Letter of Support vs Memorandum of Understanding

Letters of Support and Memorandum of Understanding overlap on various aspects. However, there are distinct features differentiating them from each other:

Characteristics	Letters of Support	Memorandum of understanding
Tone	Usually, informal	Formal
Purpose	To enhance the possibility of awarding the grant	To delineate the collaboration between the stakeholders
Content	Mentioning support for the project—May include the terms of support	Should include the terms of support—Human resources/financial/technical, etc.

Similarly, Letters of Support are different from letters of recommendation though they are provided by others in support of the applicant. Letters of recommendation are availed for the purpose of applying for fellowships and awards [7]. Contrary to Letters of Support, letters of recommendation are written by individuals who are not actively involved in the research project but are quite familiar with the qualifications and competencies of the applicant [7].

5.7 Significance of a Letter of Support

A well-written Letter of Support can act as a voice in favor of the proposal during the evaluation by the funding agencies [8]. The presence of appropriate Letters of Support will assure the funding agency that the project is in the right direction [6]. The mere presence of a letter of support do not ensure the awarding of the grant. However, Letters of Support provide an edge in highly competitive grant awards, especially when provided from highly credible and trustworthy individuals or foundations [5].

A Letter of Support can induce a sense of mutual involvement in the project between the funding agency and stakeholder providing the letter. In other words, the funding agency feels better that other credible individuals or organizations are involved in the project [10]. Further, a letter of support can also be utilized as a medium to project the requisite qualifications and competencies of the applicant in undertaking and completing the project [7].

5.8 Conclusion

The process of grant writing requires a meticulous and methodical approach by the researcher. Letters of Support can be provided by the various stakeholder/collaborators/beneficiaries of the research proposal. Letters of Support can work as a statement of commitment by individuals or agencies for accomplishing the objectives in hand with the researcher. Letters of Support can enhance the possibility of awarding grants for the research proposal.

Sample letter of support:
From,
XXX (Name),
YYY (Agency Name),

ZZZ (Complete address of the Provider)
To,
AAA (Funding agency/Representative of the funding agency)
BBB (Funding agency name),
CCC (Address of the funding agency).
Dear Mr. AAA,

It is my pleasure to write a letter in support of the project titled "..." submitted to the grant program "..." of your esteemed funding agency. (*Opening statement*)

I/We have had the opportunity to collaborate with Mr/Dr. V in the above-mentioned project with respect to ... (the relationship between the researcher and the provider of the letter) (*Middle part*)

I/We fully support the project proposed by Mr/Dr. V and his/her application for funding in your funding agency under the grant program. (*Closing/Concluding part*)

Thanking you,
Yours sincerely,
Signature
XXX (Name and designation),
YYY (Agency Name)
Seal of the institution.

Case Scenario 1

Dr. A, a young medical researcher has a proposal for studying biomarkers for suicidal behavior in individuals presenting with depression. The evaluation of biomarkers requires purchase of kits and involvement resource personnel from the clinical laboratory. The researcher has planned to obtain an extramural grant from one of the funding agencies.

A. What would be the steps in acquiring a letter of support?
B. Write a draft for requesting the letter of support from the collaborators.
C. Prepare a template for the collaborator to provide the letter of support.

Case Scenario 2

Dr. B, Professor in Psychiatry wants to study the imaging findings in schizophrenia using a functional MRI. However, the institute of the researcher does not have fMRI facility. He wants to avail the facility in an imaging center outside along with the Radiologist in his institute. Further, in order to achieve the estimated sample size, he plans to evaluate patients from various institutes and rehabilitation centers. He applies for a grant from a National Grant Agency for covering the costs of doing the imaging procedure.

A. Who all would be the potential collaborators in the project?
B. Who all can the professor approach for the Letters of Support?

References

1. Gholipour A, Lee EY, Warfield SK. The anatomy and art of writing a successful grant application: a practical step-by-step approach. Pediatr Radiol. 2014;44(12):1512–7.
2. Jacob BA, Lefgren L. The impact of research grant funding on scientific productivity. J Public Econ. 2011;95(9–10):1168–77.
3. Zlowodzki M, Jönsson A, Kregor PJ, Bhandari M. How to write a grant proposal. Indian J Orthop. 2007;41(1):23–6.
4. Sohn E. Secrets to writing a winning grant. Nature. 2020;577(7788):133–5.
5. What are grant letters of support? [Internet]. The Balance Small Business. https://www.thebalancesmb.com/what-is-a-letter-of-support-for-a-grant-proposal-2502223. Accessed 2 Dec 2021.
6. Letters of Support | NIH: National Institute of Allergy and Infectious Diseases [Internet]. https://www.niaid.nih.gov/grants-contracts/letters-of-support. Accessed 2 Dec 2021.
7. Bhosale U. Learn how to write a persuasive letter of support for grant [Internet]. Enago Academy. 2021. https://www.enago.com/academy/write-a-letter-of-support-for-grant/. Accessed 19 Jul 2022.
8. PGW Admin. What to include in a letter of support for a grant [Internet]. Professional Grant Writer. 2021. https://www.professionalgrantwriter.org/include-letter-support-grant-application. Accessed 2 Dec 2021.
9. G.400—PHS 398 Research Plan Form [Internet]. https://grants.nih.gov/grants/how-to-apply-application-guide/forms-f/general/g.400-phs-398-research-plan-form.htm#9. Accessed 2 Dec 2021.
10. Barker L, Rattihalli RR, Field D. How to write a good research grant proposal. Paediatr Child Health. 2016;26(3):105–9.

Part II

The Process for Grant Writing

Writing a Grant Proposal for a Single Centre Study: Step-by-Step Approach

Vikram Kate, Divya Gupta, and Gurushankari Balakrishnan

The journey of a 1000 miles begins with one step

Lao Tzu

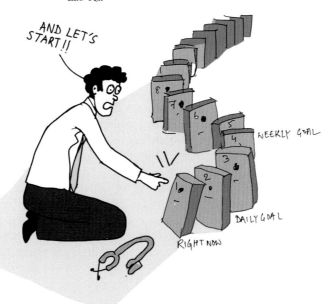

Writing a grant proposal for a single centre study-step-by-step approach

V. Kate (✉)
Department of General and Gastrointestinal surgery, Jawaharlal Institute of Postgraduate Medical Education and Research (JIPMER), Pondicherry, India

D. Gupta
Department of Dermatology, Dr. B.R. Ambedkar Medical College, Bengaluru, India

Division of Pediatric Dermatology, Manipal Hospitals, Bengaluru, India

G. Balakrishnan
Department of Surgery, Jawaharlal Institute of Postgraduate Medical Education and Research (JIPMER), Pondicherry, India

© The Author(s), under exclusive license to Springer Nature Singapore Pte Ltd. 2023
S. C. Parija, V. Kate (eds.), *Grant writing for medical and healthcare professionals*,
https://doi.org/10.1007/978-981-19-7018-4_6

Objectives
By the end of the chapter, the readers will have a good idea about
- How to respond to a call for funding
- How to define a research question for writing a grant
- Key elements of a grant proposal and how to write them
- How to prepare project timelines with the help of a Gantt Chart
- How to write the budget in a grant

6.1   Introduction

Creating an original article is one of the best experiences during any training period. Although the opportunities provided for everyone may vary but most of them have some exposure to research. Apart from the professional skills one acquires in their medical field, it is also important to ensure the development of adequate skills in scientific research. One of the important components of scientific research is acquisition of a grant for the study so that the quality of the research is uninhibited due to financial constraints and can be optimised to the highest level. Funding for a project can play an important role in executing projects, whether large or small, which require resources and facilities that are not ordinarily available at the researcher's centre. Grant writing is extremely competitive and usually less than 20% of the submitted projects are accepted for funding [1]. Most of the medical councils of various countries recommend carrying out original research at the level of trainees, junior and senior consultants both at the university affiliated and non-affiliated government and private sector hospitals. Grant writing combines one's scientific skills such as planning a study, applying appropriate statistical methods, administrative skills, and budgeting skills. The steps in writing a grant proposal are described below (Fig. 6.1).

6.2   Responding to a Call for Funding

The funding agency puts out a notice for submission of research proposals for a particular amount of money. Most funding agencies send out periodic notices (e.g. once a year) and the researcher must be on the lookout for the funding call.

6.2.1   Steps in Responding to a Funding Call

- Be aware of the various funding agencies in medicine (Table 6.1).
- Make a list of funding agencies that will support research in your field of interest. There are national research bodies for funding which one needs to be aware of, for example the National Institutes of Health (USA) [2], National Institute for Health Research (UK) [3], and the Indian Council of Medical Research (ICMR) [4]. The National Institutes of Health (NIH), USA, is the primary funding agency for

Fig. 6.1 Steps in responding
to a funding call and
submitting the grant proposal

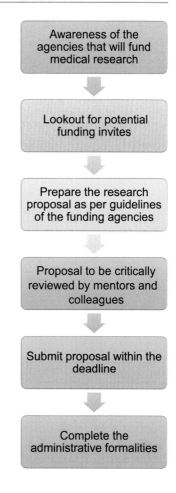

research in the field of biomedical and public health, established in 1887. The
National Institute for Health Research (NIHR), UK, is one of the largest government funding agencies in Europe for health, established in the year April 2006.
There are also specialty specific funding agencies such as the Xeroderma
Pigmentosum (XP) Society funds research in XP. The Indian Association of
Dermatologists, Venereologists and Leprologists (IADVL) funds research in
dermatology. Research specific to the field that matches the priorities of the
funding agency increases the chance of getting financed. In the era of Covid-19
pandemic, many funding agencies invited proposals to carry out research on this
virus. The very well-known Society for the Surgery of the Alimentary Tract
(SSAT), USA, offered a substantial grant for a stipulated time frame research
on Covid-19. Similarly, the Indian Council of Medical Research (ICMR) invited
proposals on Covid-19 and brought out special issues in their journal to highlight
issues on this pandemic. Similarly, there can be private organisations as well such

Table 6.1 List of Indian and international funding agencies

| Funding agencies | Indian | |
Government	Private	International
Indian Council of Medical Research Grants for • MD/MS/DM/M. Ch thesis • Post-doctoral research	Private agencies Societies for specific conditions like • Cerebral palsy • Cancer • Psoriasis • Tuberculosis • HIV-AIDS	National Institute of Health
Department of Science and Technology	Azim Premji Foundation	Bill and Melinda Gates Foundation
Department of Biotechnology	Lady Tata Memorial Trust	The Wellcome Trust
Council of Scientific and Industrial Research		Ford Foundation
National organizations of various specialties		The Rockefeller Foundation
University Grants Commission		Howard Hughes Medical Institute

MD Doctor of Medicine, *MS* Master of Surgery, *DM* Doctorate of Medicine, *M. Ch* Master of Chirurgiae, *HIV-AIDS* Human Immunodeficiency Virus-Acquired Immunodeficiency Syndrome

as CHEST Foundation, Francis Family Foundation and Burroughs Wellcome Fund [5].
- Most notices are made available on the agencies' websites. Some organisations may also put out notices in newspaper such as Council for Scientific and Industrial Research (CSIR). If the funding agency is a national or international organisation that one is part of, then the announcement may reach via email, for example, the L'Oréal Research Grant offered by the IADVL. The senior author of this chapter being a Research Committee member of the SSAT, USA, not only receives grant proposals for assessment, but he also receives invites to be disseminated among younger colleagues or trainees for funding. Colleges and institutions are other sources through which the funding call can reach the researcher.
- A good researcher will always have some projects lined up which needs funding so that the proposal can be tailored as per the funding agency guidelines and submitted within the deadline for grant application. It is necessary to read the application guidelines very carefully so that the proposal is not rejected for a relatively non-scientific reasons such as improper formatting.
- In India, studies or projects that receive foreign funding are subjected to the Foreign Contribution Regulation Act (FCRA) and must undergo an additional round of approval by the Indian regulatory authority, the HMSC (Health Ministry's Screening Committee) as well.
- A database of Indian funding agencies can be found under the Research and Development Funding Schemes of Central Government such as www.india.

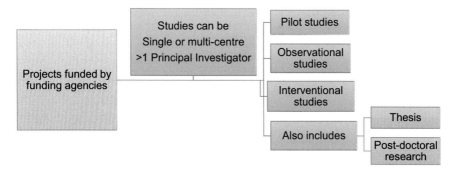

Fig. 6.2 Types of projects that can be supported by the funding agencies

gov.in or at the Research Development Office-National Centre for Biological Sciences, Tata Institute of Fundamental Research.

6.2.2 Types of Projects that can be Supported by the Funding Agencies (Fig. 6.2)

- Pilot studies.
- Observational studies.
- Interventional studies.
- Thesis.
- Post-doctoral research.
- Single-centre/Multicentric studies

6.3 Steps in Preparing the Grant Proposal

- Before we begin to write the proposal, it is important to choose the appropriate funding agencies as some of them have areas of interest in which they support work that furthers their mission. Often the topics of interest of the funding agencies are 'request for application' (RFA) document.
- Prior to writing a grant, the researcher must first define the research question. The topic must be important and relevant and must address a gap in the current knowledge in that field.
- The writer must highlight the novelty of the proposed research topic and how the result will benefit the community. The idea must lead to a significant improvement in our current medical practice or our understanding of biological processes [5]. One is unlikely to get funded for a project that does not meet the criteria. Sometimes, it is appropriate to write a proposal which may look over-ambitious, however, if satisfactorily justified, it may get an approval from the funding agencies.

- It is better to avoid too many goals in a single project especially when they are for a short-term period of 1–2 years.
- The grant application must be tailored as per the instructions of the funding agencies. Agencies have different formats and requirements, and the investigator must strictly adhere to them, including formatting, word limit and font style and size. Do not bend, modify, or get creative with the instructions. Do not hesitate in e-mailing or calling the grants agency to clarify any doubts [1].
- Whatever statements are made by the researcher in the grant application, must be supported by data or evidence to that effect. Writing style must be clear, concise and to-the-point. Avoid lengthy jargon. Spelling mistakes and grammatical errors are a strict no-no.
- When applying for a grant, if data or any previously published work on the topic from the same investigator is available, then it is good to place that in the grant proposal under the heading of 'Work already done in the field'. One need not be too modest in this section. It strengthens your proposal and makes the funding agency believe that you will be able to deliver.
- Consider collaborating with established researchers in the field. If the investigator is in the early phase of grantsmanship, and has limited experience, then associating with an established investigator can be helpful for a successful grant and will promote a good learning experience in grantsmanship.
- It is a good practice to consult a biostatistician while preparing the methodology.
- When writing the proposal, one should know that it will be reviewed by knowledgeable academic reviewers. For larger grants from many funding agencies, there is a possibility that the proposal may not be reviewed by specialists in one's field. Hence, it is necessary to make sure that the language in the proposal is not overly technical.
- Consider using flowcharts and figures to summarise the aims and methodology of the study. Time given for assessment of the proposal may vary among the reviewers and a lucid proposal with flowcharts and figures will make it easier for them to understand and review the proposal better [6].
- Any legal or ethical issues, if present, must be highlighted such as research with new drug, and research in paediatric population.
- Before submission, it is a good idea to get the proposal reviewed by senior colleagues who have prior experience in applying for grants. Soliciting inputs from colleagues and the request for a formal critique of the project plan always helps in improving the proposal.
- Avoid making a last-minute submission. Keep enough time for proof-reading, corrections, review by senior colleagues and for any technological glitches at the time of submission [1]. Rushing proposals may lead to gaping holes in the project especially in the methods or rationale which indicates inferior grantsmanship skills.

6.4   Standard Elements of a Grant Proposal

6.4.1   General Information

This is the non-scientific section and contains the personal and professional information about the principal and co-investigators. This includes name, age, address, curriculum vitae (CV), present professional responsibilities, details of other research projects currently engaged in, previous work done in the study subject, and details about the centre where the research will be conducted. Here the investigator also must describe the facilities that are required for the project, for example, technology, infrastructure, equipment, and human resource, and whether those are available at the centre. Some of the funding agencies may also require a provisional clearance from the administration about the use of the infrastructure at the centre. It should be mentioned whether it is a single department study or other specialties are also involved.

Example of a well-constructed CV or introduction to the principal researcher is 'Dr. X is a Professor of Y at Z University. He/She has a master's degree in A from B University and has more than . . . . years of experience in caring for the patients with . . . . and conducting research in this field. His/her previous research experience includes . . . (refs)'.

6.4.2   Details of the Research Project

- Cover letter: A covering letter addressed to the funding agency, with the title of the project must be submitted.
- Title page of the project: This must include the title of the project and the names and designations of the principal and the co-investigators.
- Abstract: This must describe a brief executive summary of the project and must not exceed word limit according to the guidelines, may range from 500 to 1000 words.
- Project aims and objectives: Primary and secondary objectives of the project must be mentioned. The hypotheses and objectives should be simple without much complexity so that anybody going through the proposal deciphers it clearly. An example of clear objectives is 'Eradication of H. pylori significantly reduces the relapse of duodenal ulcer after simple closure of perforation' [7]. Putting multiple, complex hypotheses may appear to be falsely impressive but can lead to the start of the proposal on a wrong foot.
- Literature review or background knowledge: This includes existing knowledge in the field and working hypothesis in the context of previous work done in the field. The significance and originality of the project must be highlighted along with the impact and benefit it is likely to have. However, it is important to tell it like a story and not like a review article. If work has been done in the past in this area, then it should be highlighted so as to demonstrate one's knowledge in the field [8]. The background should conclude in a manner that makes it obvious for the reader to

presume that the study proposal is very necessary to bridge the gap in the literature [9]. Design a win-win proposal in such a manner that whatever the outcome of the study, it will be a major addition to the literature and publishable. This also gives an impression to the reviewers that you have already thought about the future perspectives of the study. Stick to the word limit as per guidelines. This section may usually be in the range of 1000 to 1500 words.

- Project description or methodology:
  This must include:
  - Study design.
  - Sample size (including details of sample size calculation).
  - Duration of the study.
  - Study population (from whom study subjects will be drawn).
  - Study subjects: Inclusion and exclusion criteria (for both cases, and controls, if any).
  - Sampling technique and randomisation method (if applicable).
  - Method of data collection: demographic and personal data or clinical data or laboratory data.
  - Therapeutic response: Details of intervention(s) and measurement(s) of efficacy and safety of intervention(s) if any.
  - Study variables (data to be recorded to fulfil the objectives): For therapeutic studies, primary and secondary end point measurements, safety data.
  - Statistical methods: Describe in detail the methods used to present and analyse different study variables with reference to objective(s) of the study.
  - Operational definitions.
  - Limitations of the study.
- References-limited number of references must be appended at the end. The reference citation as well as the style should be in accordance with the guidelines.
- The word count for the entire proposal may vary from 2000 to 5000 words, depending on the size of the proposal and amount of grant money.

Figure 6.3 depicts the standard elements of a grant proposal.

6.4.3   Timeline of the Project

Here the investigator must mention the proposed deadlines, including project beginning date and project ending date. The project timeline and the workflow must be described in detail, preferably in a Gantt chart format [10].

A Gantt chart is a type of bar chart which shows the timeline of various milestones in any project [10]. It is an important part of project management, especially in the context of conducting any study. The vertical axis contains the list of activities, and the horizontal axis shows the time interval for each activity. The length of each bar denotes the time taken for each activity.

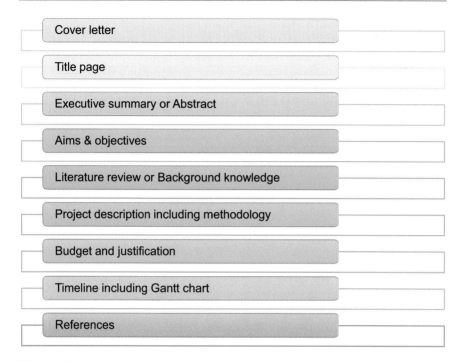

Fig. 6.3 Standard elements of a grant proposal

A Gantt chart helps in breaking up the project into specific steps with respective assigned time intervals. Each of these steps then becomes a goal that is measurable, achievable, and time bound.

6.4.4 Budgeting for a Grant

6.4.4.1 Steps in Preparing a Budget for a Grant

- Budget must be appropriate, should make sense, and should be within the grant limit.
- Initial preparation of budget can be done in a spreadsheet under different heads.
- Start by adding unit cost, followed by number of units of the required item, for the duration of the project.
- Do this for all the required items to get the sum-total, and it should be calculated so that the proposal does not lead to underfunding or overfunding of the project. Underfunding of the project can be disastrous, as there will be a dilemma about the source for additional funding to complete the project. On the contrary, an overfunded budget can raise questions with the reviewers which can lead to a potential rejection of the proposal.
- Add justification for each of the items.
- Pay close attention to the rules of purchase or recruitment.

- Avoid any mathematical errors in computing the budget.
- Avoid back-calculations in a proposal budgeting. If a complex budget ends up totalling exactly at the budget limit, the first instinct of the reviewer is to figure out how that happened and suggests that back-calculations may have occurred.

6.4.4.2 Typical Categories for Preparing a Budget are as Follows

- Recurring expenses:
  - Consumables or reagents or supplies: These are most likely to be accepted and hence must be budgeted for generously. Examples include printer ink, stationery, reagents, gloves, masks, blades, syringes, vacutainers, among other things.
  - For consumables, get the quotes from the supplier beforehand and keep it ready.
  - Personnel or staff salaries—Many projects can be managed with the support of in-house personnel such as laboratory technicians, data collectors, and stenographers. However, sometimes a particular project may need specific personnel for it. The investigator needs to justify in detail about the requirement of the staff and be very specific about their skill set as there is a possibility of rejection. Budgeting of staff must be done only for the duration of the project. One may also consider outsourcing the personnel and budget accordingly.
- Non-recurring expenses:
  - Equipment: Be specific in describing the make and model of the equipment. Maintenance cost can be added.
  - Trial insurance (if any).
  - Others: Travel, institutional overheads, ethics committee fees (if any). The travel cost should include the direct project related travel such as patient reimbursement on follow-up visits, personnel training visits if any, and the cost involved for the presentation of papers from the project at various conferences.
  - Patient re-imbursement and investigations.
  - Depending upon the place where the research project will be carried out (for example, in corporate hospitals), one may also have to factor in the Goods and Services Tax (GST) that may be levied on the grant money. It is a good idea to have one's institute's policy clarified by the finance department ahead of time.
- The above may vary from agency to agency and may depend on the project requirement. If the project is for more than a year, then specific year-wise requirement of budget must be given. If it is a multicentric study, then the budget for each centre must be provided separately.
- Budgeting for institutional overheads: Institutional overheads implies a percentage of the grant money to be paid to the institute where the study is being conducted. This is to account for the various facilities like electricity, water, vehicle, telephone, and space to conduct the study that the institute provides to the researcher. This amount may vary from 5% to as much as 20% of the grant money, depending on the setting.

6.5   Documents to be Submitted with Grant Application

- Brief CV of principal investigator.
- Brief CV of co-investigators.
- Letter of consent from Head/s of the department/s involved in the research projects (Principal investigator/s and Co-investigator/s).
- Letter of consent from the Head of the Institute where the study will be conducted.
- Undertaking duly signed by all the investigators.
- If the project requires collaboration with external agency or service provider, then, undertaking from external agency is required about expertise to hold the tests and assurance that the cost of such tests shall remain static throughout the duration of the study.

6.6   After Submission

Sometimes the grant agency may ask for clarifications, which must be addressed promptly. One must wait to hear from the agency whether the research proposal is accepted or not. If accepted, then one needs to complete the administrative formalities, like providing the bank details, where the money will be transferred.

The funding agency may ask for the following documents prior to release of the grant money
- Case record form.
- Informed consent form.
- Patient information sheet.
- Ethics committee approval from the centre.
- Registration of trials in either national or international clinical trials registry system such as Clinical Registry of India (CTRI), ClinicalTrials.gov, etc. The acknowledgement of registration needs to be submitted.
- Memorandum of Understanding (MoU) with collaborators if applicable.
- Clinical trial insurance if applicable.

6.7   If At First You Don't Succeed...

- Find out why the proposal got rejected.
- Email the agency to ask for feedback and scores. Many times, this helps in strengthening future proposals [1].
- Reviewer critiques are the roadmap to revising the proposal.
- Address every query and critique by the reviewer in resubmission.
- The response to reviewers must be presented in a lucid way so that its clear to the reviewers.
- Be persistent and try again and again.

- Anticipate rejection and be prepared for at least one resubmission to achieve a fundable score.

6.8   Carry Out the Project

The project must be carried out as proposed and must be completed within the given time frame. All the invoices must be maintained carefully for any inspection from the funding agency.

6.9   Submit a Report to the Funding Agency

Once the project is completed, a report must be submitted to the funding agency. If the project extends for more than a year, then yearly reports may have to be submitted.

6.10   Things to Keep in Mind While Writing a Grant

- Start with grants of small amounts first.
- Early career investigators can get aid from institutional grant coaching groups, when available, which can be an effective method for grant acquisition efforts [11].
- Choose a funding agency, that is likely to fund your research, for example, research in a rare genetic skin disorder epidermolysis bullosa (EB) is more likely to be funded by the Dystrophic EB Research Association (DEBRA) than by the ICMR. In the era of Covid-19 pandemic, many grant agencies were liberal for sanctioning grants in the field of Covid-19 research.
- Read the fine print—many grants do not cover salary of personnel, buying of new equipment among other things.
- Check the criterion for applying—for some grants which are provided by national associations of various specialities, only life members may be eligible. Other criteria may include nationality and age cut-offs.
- Different grants are there for different stages of one's career. For example, Burroughs Wellcome-DBT provides both early career fellowship grant as well as intermediate and senior career fellowships [5]. Separate funding is also available for post-graduate student thesis.
- Some agencies may ask whether the project has been submitted previously.
- Disclose any financial or non-financial conflicts of interest between the PI and the funder.
- Identify the limitations and mention it in the proposal to clarify it to the reviewers as they will see it anyway. It needs to be justified that these limitations will not compromise the results and interpretation.

Sometimes a good collaboration on the national or international level can allow sophisticated techniques to be used such as mutational analysis without the aid of a grant. In a study on GIST patients such mutational analysis showed the germline c.1676T>C mutation in c-kit exon 11 in the peripheral blood and a second exon 11 mutation, c.1669T>A in the tumour biopsy [12]. This shows that apart from knowledge of acquisition of a grant, collaborative effort is equally important. Although good publications can be published on clinical material, a project based on grant aid can always enrich and upgrade a clinical project and hence, whenever possible, try to target towards grant-aided projects [13, 14].

6.11 Conclusion

Writing a grant and applying for funding is a must-have skill for someone in research and academia. It allows the researcher to do good scientific work and convert his/her theories or ideas into concrete results without resource crunch. It also adds great value to one's CV. However, it is a time-consuming and challenging task, especially for first-time writers. For writing a successful grant, one needs to plan ahead, have in mind focused objectives, write in a clear and concise manner, and above all, follow one's interests. Budgeting for laboratory reagents and equipment often requires inter-departmental collaboration as clinicians may not be very well versed with these aspects. Other issues that often get overlooked are addition of GST, steep institutional overheads, and possible health ministry regulations, especially with respect to foreign funding. Beginners also benefit greatly from the inputs of mentors and previous grant recipients. To conclude, winning the funding is extremely gratifying, allows you to do the research that you want without getting encumbered about resources and yields great benefits in the long run. Hence, do not give up. Keep on writing.

Case Scenario 1
You want to write a research proposal to establish the efficacy of a new treatment Dupilumab for moderate to severe atopic dermatitis. This molecule has recently been approved by the USFDA and the European Medical Agency for use in this condition. All patients with moderate to severe atopic dermatitis, who have not responded to conventional immunosuppressive therapy will be included in this study. The improvement will be measured by using quality of life scales and associated markers like serum IgE, IL-4, and IL-13. The proposed duration of the project will be 1 year

A. Prepare a timeline for the project.
B. Prepare a budget for this project.

Case Scenario 2

Arrange in order the steps in responding to a funding call and submitting the grant proposal
A. Research proposal preparation.
B. Awareness of the agencies funding medical research.
C. Critical review by colleague.
D. Submit proposal.
E. Lookout for invites.
F. Proposal reviewed by mentor.

References

1. Sohn E. Secrets to writing a winning grant. Nature. 2020;577:133–5.
2. National Institutes of Health. https://www.nih.gov/.
3. National Institute for Health Research. https://www.nihr.ac.uk/.
4. Shi WY, Smith JA. Obtaining support and grants for research. In: Parija SC, Kate V, editors. Thesis writing for master's and Ph.D. program. Singapore: Springer Nature; 2018. p. 35–44.
5. Files DC, Hume PS, Krall J, Montemayor K, Schmidt EP, King LS. Grant writing for clinicians in training: an important career development exercise. Chest. 2020;157:932–5.
6. Ardehali H. How to write a successful grant application and research paper. Circ Res. 2014;114:1231–4.
7. Bose AC, Kate V, Ananthakrishnan N, Parija SC. *Helicobacter pylori* eradication prevents recurrence after simple closure of perforated duodenal ulcer. J Gastroenterol Hepatol. 2007;22:345–8.
8. Mohsina S, Shanmugam D, Sureshkumar S, Kundra P, Mahalakshmy T, Kate V. Adapted ERAS pathway vs. standard care in patients with perforated duodenal ulcer—a randomized controlled trial. J Gastrointest Surg. 2018;22:107–16.
9. Saurabh K, Sureshkumar S, Mohsina S, Mahalakshmy T, Kundra P, Kate V. Adapted ERAS pathway versus standard care in patients undergoing emergency small bowel surgery: a randomized controlled trial. J Gastrointest Surg. 2020;24:2077–87.
10. Li L, Roberts SC, Kulp W, Wing A, Barnes T, Colandrea N, et al. Epidemiology, infection prevention, testing data, and clinical outcomes of COVID-19 on five inpatient psychiatric units in a large academic medical center. Psychiatry Res. 2021;298:113776.
11. Weber-Main AM, McGee R, Eide Boman K, Hemming J, Hall M, Unold T, et al. Grant application outcomes for biomedical researchers who participated in the National Research Mentoring Network's Grant writing coaching programs. PLoS One. 2020;15:e0241851.
12. Gupta D, Chandrashekar L, Larizza L, Colombo EA, Fontana L, Gervasini C, et al. Familial gastrointestinal stromal tumors, lentigines, and café-au-lait macules associated with germline c-kit mutation treated with imatinib. Int J Dermatol. 2017;56:195–201.
13. Shankar H, Sureshkumar S, Gurushankari B, Sreenath GS, Kate V. Factors predicting length of stay after abdominal wall hernia repair—a prospective observational study. Turk J Surg. 2021;37:96–102.
14. Varuna S, Sureshkumar S, Gurushankari B, Archana E, Mohsina S, Kate V, et al. Association between variceal bleed and *Helicobacter pylori* infection in patients with cirrhosis with portal hypertension—a cohort study. Sultan Qaboos Univ Med J. 2021;2021:136.

Budgeting the Project: Detailing the Required Funding and Expenditure

Satish G. Patil

There is no magic in magic, it's all in the details

Walt Disney

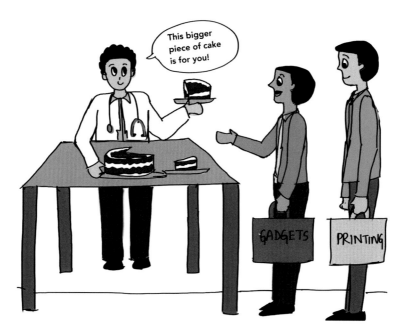

Budgeting the project-detailing the required funding and expenditure

S. G. Patil (✉)
SDM College of Medical Sciences and Hospital, Shri Dharmasthala Manjunatheshwara University, Dharwad, Karnataka, India

S. C. Parija, V. Kate (eds.), *Grant writing for medical and healthcare professionals*, https://doi.org/10.1007/978-981-19-7018-4_7

Objectives
- Understand the various components of a budget proposal
- Realize the various types of costs to be mentioned in a budget proposal

7.1 Introduction

Financial support is essential for carrying out any research. Budgeting for a research project is one of the key elements of grant writing. A budget is a quantitative expression of a financial plan for the expenses to be incurred on the project during the proposed period of time. The budget plan demonstrates the cost required for carrying out the project, forecasts the expenditure for a particular purpose in detail, and serves the sponsors a financial plan of how the grantee organization will spend the money on the proposed research project. The budget plan depicts the funders, exactly what and how much they can support, and where their fund will be used upon the release of the grant. Also, it will help the awardee organization and the investigators in managing the project. Most importantly, a budget plan for the project is crucial for accountability [1].

A full understanding of planning and preparing a project budget is essential for estimating and detailing the required expenses. The proposed budget should clearly convince the grant reviewers about the cost expenditure and need for funds. It is important to keep in mind that the grant reviewers will note both over and under the projection of the expenses [2]. This chapter provides insights on estimating, planning, and writing a budget for research grants. Keeping in view the variability in the components of the budget and projection of the expenses (to be incurred for the proposed project) among the funding organizations, it has been endeavored to explain all the types of costs used in the grant funding (India, USA, UK, Europe, and others).

7.2 Main Types of Project Costs

The project costs can be divided into several ways. The most common methods used for categorizing a budget for a research project are as follows [3–6]:

1. **Direct and indirect costs**: Direct costs are the expenses incurred specifically to carry out a project which include costs towards human resources, instruments, materials or consumables, and travel. Indirect costs are the expenses required to run a project, but they are not directly attributed to the specific expenses of a project. Indirect costs are the overhead charges which include facilities provided by the institution to run a proposed research project such as hospital, medical records, laboratory, electricity, water, and library.
2. **Fixed and variable costs:** Fixed costs are the expenses that remain the same throughout the research project, such as rent, laboratory, or institutional charges.

Variable costs are the expenses that change with the amount of research work carried out during the study period. These costs are incurred for chemicals, diagnostic kits, stationeries, animals, and patients/participants.

3. **Recurring and non-recurring costs:** Recurring costs are the variable expenses that keep on occurring during the entire project duration. Budget categorized for recurring expenses are the expenses incurred for the items such as experimental animals, consumables, chemicals, glassware, diagnostic kits, stationeries (books, pens, prints, photocopies), communication (mailing, telephone, internet), survey materials (tools, questionnaires), publication, reprints, investigations (biochemical, clinical, radiological), physician or consultant fees, food charges, research patient allowances, and salary and wages of personnel. Non-recurring costs are the one-time expenses incurred during the study period of the particular project. These expenses do not recur or are required again and again while running a research project. The budget categorized for non-recurring expenses is the costs incurred for equipment or instruments, accessories of equipment, computer, and printers, application software(s), electrical and electronic items, etc. The allowable cost and limits for the non-recurring budget may vary among several funding organizations or agencies. Few funding agencies may allocate their maximum budget for non-recurring expenses which help in the development of infrastructure and establishment/upgradation of the laboratory.

7.3   Components of Project Budget

The research project budget may consist of the following parts [7]
1. **Personnel:** If the study requires human resources, then the budget for personnel can be listed in this section by their role in the project.
   (a) **Salary:** The salary for the staff with different designations varies from sponsor to sponsor. Salaries with allowances for the personnel can be budgeted as per the guidelines of the funding agency. The salary for the principal and co-investigators may or may not be allowable. The funding agency determines and fixes the budget as the salary amount for the personnel working in the project at different capacities or designations. National Institute of Health (NIH) grant determines the salary and fringe benefits based on the institutional base salary and the amount of time or effort (person-months) devoted by the investigator to the project. The amount funded as a salary amount for the project personnel may not be uniform always or throughout the duration of the project. If the proposed study requires multiple people with the same role, for example "site managers" or "public health workers," add the salaries together for that particular role or post. The salaries for the administrators or clerks or mentors may not be allowed as direct costs.
   (b) **Person-months**: Person-months or human efforts or efforts are the metrics for expressing the amount of time (or effort) devoted to the specific project

by the investigators, faculty, research fellows, assistants, or other senior personnel. The person-months is calculated by multiplying the percentage of effort devoted to the research project times the number of months of regular payment from the employer. For example, if the investigator is receiving regular payment for 12 months and will devote 12 months at 25% effort/time then the person-months equals 3 ($12 \times 0.25 = 3$). Person-months can be calculated easily using the Excel-based person-months conversion calculator developed by the National Institute of Health grants and funding, available at nexus.od.nih.gov.

(c) **Fringe benefits**: Fringe benefits are the extra benefit supplementing an employee's salary, such as healthcare facility, accommodation, and pension. Fringe benefits are budgeted as per the policy of an institution or sponsor.

(d) **Type of staff required:** The type and number of staff required depend on the amount of work in the project, the type of the study, and the number of study centers. Based on the objectives of the research and the role of the staff in the study, the organization can ask for any staff, for example, including research associate, post-doctoral fellow, senior research fellow (SRF) or junior research fellow (JRF), research assistant, laboratory technician, public health worker, attender, etc. Multicenter clinical trials or large population-based surveys may need more staff of the same cadre (based on the number of study sites) such as site investigators, site managers or site coordinators, nurses, consultants or physicians, exercise or yoga instructors, public health assistants, pharmacists, and data-entry operators.

2. **Equipment:** If the proposed research requires new equipment to carry out a project work, then a budget for the instrument(s) can be listed in this section. The annual maintenance cost of the new equipment for the proposed period of the research could also be added to this category. The equipment is usually purchased once during the research grant period; hence, it is categorized as a non-recurring budget (given below). The percentage of budget allocated (from the grant funds) for the purchase of equipment for the research may vary among the funding organizations. The equipment procured from the grant funds usually vests in the grantee institute/organization. However, after completion of the research project, the funding organization keeps the right to transfer the equipment (purchased with grant funds) to another eligible party or to the new grantee organization to continue the research using the same equipment. The equipment may also need to be shared with other grant awardees. If the equipment is not required for a longer period to continue research or the cost of equipment(s) is too high beyond the granted limit, then it can be borrowed on lease or rent. Prior approval for the purchase of equipment with grant funds may be required. Any change in the specifications of the instrument to be procured with grant funds requires prior approval from the funding organization. The title to the equipment purchased with grant funds will remain with the original grantee organization, even if the principal investigator (PI) moves to another organization, provided

the grantee organization could continue the research project with an alternate principal investigator or co-investigator.

3. **Travel costs:** Travel costs incurred for scientific meetings, conferences, workshops or training, data collection, interviews of study participants or patients, fieldwork, grant meeting, study site monitoring and auditing, travel for consultation, etc. can be budged in this section. The budget for travel should be within the allowable travel cost and limits of the sponsoring organization. For example, the budget for foreign traveling for attending or presenting the paper at scientific conferences or for undergoing training may not be uniform or allowable by all the funding organizations. The costs incurred for food and accommodation associated with travel would also be requested in the travel budget category.

4. **Registration fees for symposiums and seminars:** The registration fees for conferences, symposiums, and seminars within or outside the country can be budgeted in this category if it is allowable.

5. **Trainee costs:** Several projects, particularly multicenter clinical trials or large population-based surveys need training of project staff for uniform execution of research projects as per the study protocol. Costs incurred for personnel training on study-related procedures, such as obtaining and documenting informed consent from research participants, randomization, blinding, allocation concealment, intervention protocol, data collection, and data entry, interviewing techniques for data collection, trial documentation, animal or laboratory experimental skills, and surgical skills, are provisioned to be budgeted in the trainee expenses.

6. **Contingency or materials and supplies:** The costs incurred for consumables, office supplies specifically for the project, laboratory materials, glassware, chemicals, electronic and electrical items, animals and animal care, communications, stationeries, test materials or samples, questionnaire forms, data access, report materials, prints, and photocopies, etc. can be budgeted as contingency or consumables or materials and supplies.

7. **Consultant services:** The budget in this category will be used for consultant (s) services. They support the project but do not involve directly in the execution of the project. The consultants are those individuals who will provide training (animal handling and experiments, special experimental techniques, instrumentation, equipment operation, etc.) to the project staff, clinical or physician services (examination of research patients), and advice (experts advice, legal advice) to the project; help in the development of a tool, questionnaire, exercise or yoga or meditation programs, software applications, web-designing, implementation strategy in implementation research, data analysis plan, etc. Consultant service can also be hired for the analysis of the data of the project as a third party, patenting and copyright filing, auditing, and others as per the requirement of the proposed project. The budget for services taken from a consulting firm would also be requested in this category.

8. **Publication costs:** The article processing fee (APC), open access fee and other costs associated with the publication of research findings in a journal could be budgeted if it is allowable in the grant funds.

9. **Facilities and administrative (F & A) costs:** Formerly known as indirect costs are the costs incurred in conducting or supporting research and service, but they are not directly attributed to the specific expenses of a project. Indirect costs are termed as F & A costs (NIH grant fund) or overhead charges (other grant funds). Facilities costs are incurred in supporting activities such as plant operation and maintenance (utilities, routine maintenance, repairs, etc.), depreciation or use allowance (for buildings and equipment), and library expenses (books, library staff, etc.). Administrative costs are incurred in supporting activities such as general administration (accounting, administrative offices, clerks, auditing, etc.), sponsored project administration (other personnel and costs of offices involved in the administration of sponsored projects), departmental administration expenses (administrative costs at the Institute/departmental levels), and student administration or services. F & A rate is calculated by dividing the F & A cost incurred for research conducted during the selected year by the direct costs (salaries, fringe benefits, materials and supplies, travel, etc.) during that year.

10. **Overhead costs:** Overhead charges are the costs (indirect costs) which include facilities provided by the research center/college to run a proposed research project such as hospital, medical records, laboratory, electricity, water, and library. It is calculated by multiplying the sponsor's overhead rate (usually fixed) with the direct costs. A fixed cost of about 5–15% of the total budget (excluding the cost for equipment) is provisioned as an institutional overhead cost that goes to the institution for supporting research. For example, if the total budget for the proposed research is 50 Lakhs including equipment cost of 6 Lakhs, then the overhead costs (if 10%) equals 4.6 Lakhs ($50 - 6 = 46 \times 0.1$).

11. **In-kind costs or contributions:** In-kind contributions are the services or goods or materials received at a conservative value for the project. For example, goods or services provided instead of cash for the project or professional services such as legal, accounting, and medical at a customary hourly rate. These are the items or services provided for the project that otherwise be paid from the project budget.

12. **Other costs:** The costs incurred for other services or items can be budgeted such as for research patient care (including travel and daily allowances), alterations and renovations, computer services, purchase of books and articles or journals and periodicals, printing pamphlets, advertisements, patient reimbursements, insurance, and hospitalization.

13. **Modified total direct cost (MTDC):** Modified total direct cost is the base to which the indirect costs or facilities and administrative rates (F & A) are applied. It includes salaries and fringe benefits, materials and supplies, travel, and services. It excludes equipment costs, patient care costs, participant support costs, rental costs, scholarships or fellowships, and tuition-related fees.

14. **Modular and detailed grant budget:** The direct costs of the grant budget are requested in specific modules (or increments) in the modular budget. And in a detailed budget, the direct costs are requested in detailed line items. For example, the total direct costs in the detailed budget are divided by a number of years and rounded up into modules (such as 25,000 USD or 50,000 USD).

7.4 Detailing the Required Funding and Expenditure with Justification

Detailing the required budget is a line-item representation of the expenses (year-wise) to be incurred for the proposed project. The budget justification includes in-depth detailing of the line-items costs with the purpose of requirement and utilization. The detailed budget with justification is nothing but a budget narrative.

Each line item added to the budget in different categories must be justified separately. An example includes the need for consultants or experts, or equipment for the proposed project because of unavailability within the awardee organization. The need for human resources with their role in the project, the need for attending conferences or meetings, purchase of periodicals or books should be explained and justified [8].

The budget should be prepared in consultation with the experts and administrators. Get confirmed about the cost of items from at least two to three suppliers or distributors before putting the estimates in the budget. The cost estimates for each line item should be as accurate as possible because both over-estimation and under-estimation are looked at suspiciously by the reviewers [9].

To make it easier to understand the process of detailed budgeting, an overview of the budget system of two funding organizations is shown in Tables 7.1 and 7.2, respectively. These sample budgets will help in planning and writing budgets for most of the grants (particularly, on health research) worldwide. Each category with a line-item added (as an example) in the two sample budgets with sample calculations is explained below in detail (refer to pages no. 7–9). The line-item budget is typically divided into either direct costs (personnel, equipment, consumables, materials and supplies, travel, services) and indirect costs (overhead charges or F & A charges) or recurring (personnel, consumables/contingency, travel), non-recurring (equipment and accessories) and indirect costs. Several expenses might arise other than the above-mentioned typical budget categories which can be budgeted in other costs categories. Remember, the budget in each category should be clearly understandable to the reviewers, that's why the particular item is added, the cost estimates of each item, and how the sub-totals of the expenses for each category are reached.

Any year-wise variation in the line items should be described in the budget justification. For example, the salary for the staff may be needed only for the first 2 years or the last 2 years, or the amount has been kept aside for the third year for consultants who help in the analysis and interpretation of data. If the participant recruitment will be more in the second year, then more funds for consumables or participant costs may be allocated for the second-year budget (refer to Table 7.2).

Table 7.1 Sample of detailed budget-1

| 1. Salaries (A & B) | | | | | | | | Year-1: Period 2021–2022 |
Name	Role	Type of appointment (9/10/12 month)	% Effort	Summer months	Base salary (USD)	Salary requested (USD)	Fringe benefit (USD)	Total
A. Senior/key person								
Mr. XXX	Lead PI	9	25%	–	100,000	25,000	8000	33,000
Ms. YYY	Co-PI	12	15%	–	90,000	13,500	4320	17,820
Mr. ZZZ	Co-PI	10	15%		90,000	13,500	4320	17,820
B. Other personnel								
Mr. AAA	Research coordinator	–	100%	–	35,000	35,000	11,200	46,200
Ms. BBB	Yoga instructor	–	100%	–	25,000	25,000	8000	33,000
Mr. CCC	Graduate (2)		–	3	5000	10,000	845	10,845
Ms. DDD	Lab technician	12	60%	–	15,000	9000	2880	11,880
Mr. EEE	Data entry clerk	12	50%	–	15,000	7500	2400	9900
Total salary and wages						138,500	41,965	**180,465**
2. Equipment								
Equipment A	Noninvasive vascular analyzer							8500
Equipment B	Noninvasive endothelial function testing device							6000
Sub-total								**14,500**
3. Travel								
Domestic								5500
International								0

4. Supplies and materials	
Project-specific office supplies and postage	2500
Food supplies	3500
Educational supplies	1000
Data processing supplies	4800
Medical supplies	12,000
Subtotal	**23,800**
5. Other direct costs	
Participant costs	1100
Consultations	4450
Training costs	0
ADP/computer services	0
Alterations and renovations	500
Printing	2700
Publication costs	6000
Subtotal	**14,750**
Subtotal direct costs	**239,015**
Subcontracts	0
MTDC (modified total direct cost)	**209,765**
6. Indirect costs	
F & A rate (8% × MTDC)	**16,781**
Total direct and indirect costs	**255,796**

Table 7.2 Sample detailed budget-2

Item		Budget (in Rupees)			
		1st Year	2nd Year	3rd Year	Total
A. Recurring					
1. Budget for salaries/wages					
Designation and number of persons	*Monthly emoluments*	INR	INR	INR	INR
Junior research fellow [4]	27,500 (25,000 + 10% HRA) × 4	13,20,000	13,20,000	13,20,000	39,60,000
Research assistant [1]	16,500 (15,000 + 10% HRA) × 4	1,98,000	1,98,000	1,98,000	5,94,000
Yoga instructors [4]	16,500 (15,000 + 10% HRA) × 4	7,92,000	7,92,000	–	15,84,000
Sub-total		23,10,000	23,10,000	15,18,000	61,38,000
2. Budget for consumable materials					
ECG electrodes, glassware, chemicals		6000	6000	6000	18,000
Commercial diagnostic kits		60,000	60,000	60,000	1,80,000
Data acquisition charges from web-portal (cloud) related to ambulatory BP data		30,000	30,000	30,000	90,000
Sub-total		96,000	96,000	96,000	2,88,000
3. Budget for travel					
Travel for PI and Co-I		15,000	15,000	15,000	45,000
Travel for training		42,000	–	–	42,000
Travel for site visits		84,000	42,000	42,000	1,68,000
Travel for investigators meeting		42,000	42,000	42,000	1,26,000
Inland travel for conferences attending and presentation		–	15,000	15,000	30,000
Sub-total		1,83,000	1,14,000	1,14,000	4,11,000
4. Budget for contingencies					
Stationeries/photocopying/postage/printing/report printing		12,000	12,000	12,000	36,000
Sub-total		12,000	12,000	12,000	36,000
5. Other costs					
Publication expenses (journals)		–	50,000	50,000	1,00,000
B. Equipment		0	0	0	0
Total direct costs (A + B)		26,01,000	25,82,000	17,90,000	69,73,000
C. Overhead cost (indirect costs)					
(Total direct costs-equipment cost) × 5%		1,30,050	1,29,100	89,500	3,48,650
Grand total (A + B + C)		27,31,050	27,11,100	18,79,500	73,21,650

7.4.1   Sample Budget-1: Budget Justifications and Sample Calculation (Table 7.1)

This sample (National Institute of Health grants, USA) shows a budget estimate for 1 year only (Table 7.1). The line-item budgets are typically divided into direct costs (personnel, equipment, materials and supplies, travel, and other direct costs) and indirect costs (F & A charges). Note that the tabulated items and cost estimates are for examples, to be used for guidelines/reference only.

1. **Salaries (A & B):** The salary and wages estimate for the personnel for NIH grants is based on three factors: type of appointment, base salary, and percent of effort (amount of time devoted) for the proposed project. Type of appointment means, for how many months the salary is paid to an employee regularly: 9/10/12 months. The person-month is calculated by multiplying the percentage of effort devoted by the staff for the research project times the number of months of regular payment from the employer. For example, the person-month for the lead PI equals 2.25 (9 × 25%), for two Co-PI equals 1.8 and 1.5 (12 × 15%; 10 × 15%), respectively, and data entry clerk equals 6 (12 × 50%). The role of each line-staff (type and amount of work done) in the proposed project and their salary estimation should be described. Below, the role of staff is not explained (which needs to be specified), only sample calculations are shown for each line of staff. Base salary and fringe benefits vary among institutions or universities. So, refer to the sponsor guidelines thoroughly before calculating the estimates for salary and wages.
   (a) **Senior/Key personnel:**
      - Mr. XXX (Lead PI): Salary requested is $25,000 (Base salary × effort%: 100,000 × 25%). Fringe benefits requested is $8000 (salary requested × 32%: 25,000 × 32%). The total salary and wages requested for Mr. XXX is $33,000 (Salary + fringe benefit: 25,000 + 8000) for first year.
      - Ms. YYY (Co PI): Salary requested is $13,500 (Base salary × effort%: 90,000 × 15%). Fringe benefits requested is $4320 (salary requested × 32%: 13,500 × 32%). The total salary and wages requested for Mr. YYY is $17,820 (Salary + fringe benefit: 13,500+ 4320) for first year.
      - Ms. ZZZ (Co PI): Salary requested is $13,500 (Base salary × effort%: 90,000 × 15%). Fringe benefits requested is $4320 (salary requested × 32%: 13,500 × 32%). The total salary and wages requested for Mr. ZZZ is $17,820 (Salary + fringe benefit: 13,500+ 4320) for first year.
   (b) **Other personnel:**
      - Mr. AAA (Research coordinator): Salary requested is $35,000 (Base salary × effort%: 35,000 × 100%). Fringe benefits requested is $11,200 (salary requested × 32%: 35,000 × 32%). The total salary and wages requested for Mr. AAA is $46,200 (Salary + fringe benefit: 35,000+ 11,200) for first year.
      - Mr. BBB (Yoga instructor): Salary requested is $25,000 (Base salary × effort%: 25,000 × 100%). Fringe benefits requested is $8000 (salary

requested × 32%: 25,000 × 32%). The total salary and wages requested for Mr. BBB is $33,000 (Salary + fringe benefit: 25,000+ 8000) for first year.

- Mr. CCC (Graduate): Salary requested is $5000 for each graduate for three summer months. For two graduates: 5000 × 2 = $10,000. Fringe benefits requested is $845 (salary requested × 32%: 10,000 × 32%). The total salary and wages requested for two graduates is $10,845 (Salary + fringe benefit: 10,845 + 845) for first year.
- Ms. DDD (Lab technician): Salary requested: $15,000 × 60% (Base salary × effort%) = $9000. Fringe benefits: 9000 × 32% (salary requested × 32%) = $2880. The total salary and wages requested for Mr. DDD is $11,880 (Salary + fringe benefit: 9000 + 2880) for first year.
- Mr. EEE (Data entry clerk): Salary requested: $15,000 × 50% (Base salary × effort%) = $7500. Fringe benefits: $7500 × 32% (salary requested × 32%) = $2400. The total salary and wages requested for Mr. EEE is $9900 (Salary + fringe benefit: 7500 + 2400) for first year.

2. **Equipment:** One should ask for equipment if it is unavailable in your organization. Justify the need and utility of the requested instrument. Clearly specify the cost estimate including service tax and maintenance, if applicable.

3. **Travel:** Specify the purpose of travel. Cost for domestic travel is calculated by multiplying the cost for each travel per staff with a number of travel (3 @ $1500 per travel = $4500 + 1@ $1000 per travel).

4. **Supplies and materials:** A sample cost estimate for each line item has been mentioned in the table. Clearly specify the need for supplies and materials, indicate the items and how the cost estimate for the expenses is reached for project-specific office supplies and postage, food supplies, educational supplies, data processing supplies, and medical supplies.

5. **Other direct costs:** Calculate the expenses to be incurred for each research participant then multiply it by the number of participants required for the proposed project and estimate the total cost for participants. Cost estimate for consultation is $4450 (Mr XYZ 4 days @ $350 per day; also $1500 for travel, accommodations, and per diem) and Mr. ABC (5 days @ $250 per day). Similarly, calculate the cost and specify the expenses for training, alterations and renovations, publications, printing as per your project proposal.

6. **Indirect costs:** Modified total direct cost equals $209,765 [$29,250 (equipment cost + other direct costs) - $239,015 (sub-total direct costs)]. F & A rate for foreign organizations is 8%. So, indirect cost equals $16,781 (MTDC × F & A rate: $209,765 × 8% = $16,781).

7.4.2 Sample Budget-2: Budget Justifications and Sample Calculation (Table 7.2)

This sample (Research grants, India) shows a year-wise budget estimate for 3 years for a multicenter study (Table 7.2). The line-item budgets are typically divided into recurring costs, equipment costs (non-recurring costs), and overhead costs (indirect costs). Note that the tabulated items and cost estimates are for examples, to be used for guidelines/reference only.

1. **Recurring costs**
   (a) **Budget for salaries/wages:** The salary and wages estimate for the personnel for the Indian research grants is usually fixed by the funding organizations. Refer to the guidelines of the sponsor to know the salaries fixed for the personnel with different cadres or designations. In the above sample, the requirement of 9 staff (four junior research fellows, one research assistant, and four yoga instructors) has been indicated. Justify, why there is a requirement of 9 staff and what role they are going to play in the proposed project. For example, the study will be conducted in four sites, therefore four staff with two cadres or designations and one staff at the coordination center; a total of 9 staff is needed. Specify the criteria for selection of each staff, for example, a candidate with post-graduation in biological or medical sciences will be preferred for a junior research fellow (JRF), a graduate for a research assistant, and a graduate in yoga and naturopathy for yoga instructor post. Below, the job description of the staff associated with the project is not explained (which needs to be specified), only sample calculations are shown for each line staff.
      - **Salary for junior research fellow** (JRF): The monthly emolument for a JRF is Rs. 25,000. House rent allowance is 10% (Tier-3 city) of the monthly salary ($25,000 \times 10\% = 2500$). Therefore, salary for each JRF equals 27,500 ($25,000 + 2500 = 27,500$). The total salary needed for four JRF for each year equals Rs. 13,20,000 ($27,500 \times 12 \times 4 = 13,20,000$).
      - **Salary for research assistant:** The monthly emolument for a research assistant is Rs. 15,000. House rent allowance is 10% (Tier-3 city) of the monthly salary ($15,000 \times 10\% = 1500$). Therefore, salary for a research assistant equals 16,500 ($15,000 + 1500 = 16,500$). The total salary needed for each year equals Rs. 1,98,000 ($16,500 \times 12 = 1,98,000$).
      - **Salary for yoga instructors:** The monthly emolument for a yoga instructor is Rs. 15,000. House rent allowance is 10% (Tier-3 city) of the monthly salary ($15,000 \times 10\% = 1500$). Therefore, salary for each yoga instructor equals Rs. 16,500 ($15,000 + 1500 = 16,500$). The total salary needed for four yoga instructors for each year equals Rs. 7,92,000 ($16,500 \times 12 \times 4 = 7,92,000$). Here the salary is budgeted for the first 2 years only because of the expected completion of participant recruitment and intervention in the first 2 years (an example for readers).
   (b) **Budget for consumable materials:** Make a list of required consumables associated with the proposed project. Estimate the cost of each item. Break down the budget into item-wise and year-wise with cost calculation. An example includes a cost estimate for disposable ECG electrodes, glassware, and chemicals are Rs. 6000 per year, for diagnostic kits is Rs. 60,000 per year (utility of the kits must be specified) and for data acquisition is Rs. 30,000 per year (purpose of data acquisition must be specified).

(c) **Budget for travel:** Specify the purpose of travel. Cost for domestic travel is calculated by multiplying the cost for each travel per staff with the number of travel [(2 @ Rs. 7500 per travel = 15,000) + (travel for training: 4 @ Rs. 6500 per travel +4 @ Rs. 1000 per accommodation) + (4 visits twice in year to each site, 4 @ Rs. 6500 per travel +4 @ Rs. 1000 per accommodation), etc. The cost estimate should be on the basis of the allowable mode of travel.

(d) **Budget for contingencies:** Make a list of expenses for stationeries, photocopying, postage, the printing of data collection forms, consent forms, reports, and communication to be incurred for the project for all the sites of study. The cost estimate of all contingencies should be specified appropriately. Cost estimate for contingency equals Rs. 12,000 (Rs. 4000 per study site $\times$ 4 = 12,000).

(e) **Other costs:** The cost estimate for the article processing and publication of the research findings in a journal of repute is Rs. 1,00,000 (Rs. 50,000 per year $\times$ 2 years) from the second year onwards.

2. **Equipment costs:** If new equipment is not needed for your proposed project from the grant fund, then just mention that the facilities or instrument necessary for the project is available in your organization.

3. **Overhead costs:** 5% of the total direct costs excluding equipment cost equals Rs. 3,48,650 (69,73,000 $\times$ 5% = 3,48,650).

7.5   Conclusion

To conclude, the grant applicant needs to understand the expectations of the sponsor, read the instructions carefully and go through the budget template. Check the budget specifications and limitations, allowable and non-allowable costs. Categorize each line item as per the sponsor instructions and template.

Estimate the expenses to be incurred for each line item for each year. Break down the budget into item-wise and year-wise with cost calculation. Ensure costs are reasonable, allowable, and related to the proposed project. Justify the need for each line item associated with the project. The budget in each category should be clearly understandable to the reviewers, that why the particular item is added and how the expenses for each category are reached.

Review the budget to verify the cost estimates and calculation of expenses. It is better, if the budget is reviewed by experts and administrators or external members. Both over-and-under projections of the expenses are noted suspiciously by the grant reviewers, resulting in an increased chance of rejection.

Case Scenario
A researcher is aimed to conduct a randomized controlled trial of safety and effectiveness of yoga-based cardiac rehabilitation program on patients with coronary artery disease. The objective of the study is to determine, if yoga-based rehabilitation program can improve the cardiovascular function, functional exercise capacity, and

the quality of life. This multicenter study includes two arm, parallel, open label, randomized-controlled design.

1. What are the different types of costs in a project?
2. Enumerate the various components of a budget.

References

1. Patil SG. How to plan and write a budget for research grant proposal? J Ayurveda Integr Med. 2019;10(2):139–42.
2. How to apply—application guide | grants.nih.gov [Internet]. https://grants.nih.gov/grants/how-to-apply-application-guide.html. Accessed 11 Sept 2021.
3. Budget and cost resources [internet]. ORSP. https://orsp.umich.edu/develop-proposal/budget-and-cost-resources. Accessed 09 Aug 2021.
4. Research proposals—budget [Internet]. ORSP. https://orsp.umich.edu/research-proposals-budget. Accessed 09 Aug 2021.
5. Developing a budget. Illinois Institute of Technology: [Internet]. https://research.iit.edu/osrp/developing-budget. Accessed 09 Oct 2021.
6. India Alliance—Advancing Discovery and Innovation to Improve Health. https://www.indiaalliance.org/fellowshiptype/basic-biomedical-research-fellowships. Accessed 09 Oct 2021.
7. Revision of emoluments and guidelines on service conditions for research personnel engaged in R & D programme of the Central Government Departments/Agencies: Department of Science and Technology. https://dst.gov.in/news/revision-emoluments-and-guidelines-service-conditions-research-personnel-engaged-r-d-programme. Accessed 09 Oct 2021.
8. Indian Council for Medical Research Guidelines for Extramural Research Programme. Indian Council for Medical Research. https://main.icmr.nic.in/sites/default/files/extramural/Extramural_Projects_Guidelines.pdf. Accessed 09 Oct 2021.
9. Vision Group on Science and Technology (VGST). Guidelines and format for proposal submission [internet]. VGST/K-FIST. http://vgst.in/kfistguidelines.php. Accessed 09 Oct 2021.

Proving the Competency of the Researcher and the Adequacy of the Infrastructure to Carry Out the Research

Shree Lakshmi Devi Singaravelu

Success demands a high level of logistical and organizational competence

George S. Patton Jr.

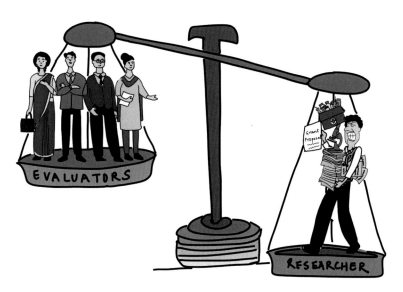

Proving the competency of the researcher and the adequacy of the infrastructure to carry out the research

S. L. D. Singaravelu (✉)
Shri Sathya Sai Medical College and Research Institute, Sri Balaji Vidyapeeth, Chengalpet, Tamil Nadu, India

S. C. Parija, V. Kate (eds.), *Grant writing for medical and healthcare professionals*,
https://doi.org/10.1007/978-981-19-7018-4_8

Objectives
- To understand the methods of providing competencies for a researcher and developing an adequate research environment.
- To identify the challenges in providing adequate infrastructure and various models to evaluate the adequacy of research infrastructure in an organization.

8.1   Good Researcher

A researcher is a loco pilot of innovative medicine. A demanding need for global standard treatment has increased the need for high-quality research. The mushrooming of doctors and health scientists has questioned the quality of researchers all over the scientific grounds. There are some basic necessitates being fulfilled by a researcher to conduct a significant and reliable research study. A good researcher must be enthusiastic to keep him/her updated on the current community need. Must adopt critical thinking and reflective thinking. A researcher should be a meticulous person with prime focus and commitment to the field of interest. A good researcher must be able to work as a team without conflict and support his peer members to achieve a common goal. An update in-field knowledge can be attained by attending regular conferences and exchanging ideas with researchers in similar fields. A current researcher must be updated with all research tools and methodologies in his expertise. The researcher should be aware of basic statistics to interpret and appraise a literature result. A good researcher must be unbiased in publishing his results even if it is negative or do not support the hypothesis. A researcher should never falsify, fabricate, or plagiarize any data as it may mislead future researchers and result in erroneous evidence-based medicine practice [1].

8.2   Competencies of a Researcher

A successful research outcome is directly dependent on the competencies one develops during the course of research life. Commonly the terms skill and competencies are bewildered. Research skills can be acquainted by training like data collection, using equipment etc., whereas competencies are abilities a researcher requires to possess to perform research. In other words, competencies have three different facets such as skill, knowledge, and abilities.

The professional competencies of a researcher are [2]
1. Cognitive skills: This is the basis of all researchers or aspiring learners. The skill targets thinking, learning, attention, perception, memory, logical reasoning, and judgement. These are the essential skills for a researcher to develop a hypothesis, a research design and select an apt methodology and implement it.
2. Communication skills: Communication with colleagues and team head and negotiation in a multicultural environment are preferred skills. A researcher needs effective communication to lead or be a part of a team. Special abilities

like quick problem solving, and decision-making should be practiced to improve response from all research stakeholders and for a good professional reputation.

3. Organizational skill: In a developing country, managing the research resource efficiently is of utmost importance and organizational skills help the researcher to utilize the resources effectively and efficiently. Researchers are multitasking personals and training in organizational skills helps them to effectively manage time, and balance between clinical duties, medical education, and research. Prioritizing and record keeping will help to recognize important goals and to arrange the tasks in a logical order for acclimatizing and tailoring the existing plan. Record keeping will improvize in knowing what is completed and the future achievements to be executed in a time-bound manner.

4. Interpersonal skills: Multidisciplinary research team always consists of diverse members committed to a common goal [3]. Interpersonal skills help to increase emotional commitment. Learning to appreciate peer team members will further strengthen the teamwork and avoid conflict among collaborative team members.

5. Competencies to manage complex teams both national and international: Communication and negotiation skills will help the researcher achieve the competency to manage both national and international teams.

6. Leadership skills: In this digital era, talented research members always look towards a work environment with guidance, support, empathy, and compassion. A good team leader should lead the team without conflict provide equal opportunity to all and appreciate and motivate the team. A leader should be a good listener and provide an ego-free fun-filled work desk for all team members [4].

7. Competencies to adapt to unfamiliar situations: A researcher will have to continuously meet new members of a team and work in a new environment for all types of collaborative research. Hence adapting to the new environment and members is the most important skill one has to acquire [5].

8.3   Providing the Competencies for the Researcher

8.3.1   The Role of an Organization

The organization should support research promoting activities on the campus. The main focus should be training the researchers to enhance basic research skills like developing research ideas, writing research protocol, applying for research grants, and publishing an article, poster, or podium presentation. To support the growth of individual researchers and follow the outcome. An organization should provide adequate direction for a career in research which will motivate young minds to pursue research and develop their research career. Regular workshops to improve communication skills and interpersonal skills will guide the researchers to take more collaborative research.

Researcher in the due course of their experience learns various research skills, but special competencies are always neglected. Programs targeting special competencies like leadership skills, conflict management, and team management will create efficient research.

8.3.2   The Role of a Researcher

The researcher must be motivated and enthusiastic to learn. Discussion with the team researcher on discussions and conclusion is crucial. Hence one should be free of conflict and self-conceit. The researcher should analyze the need of the program and organize faculty development programs. Collaborative research should be taken for integrated research. Multidisciplinary research should be amplified to provide adequate training for junior researchers.

Learning in research is multidimensional and should be incorporated at various levels by multichannel. Research learning is a mammoth process and before in-cooperating, with the junior researchers, it should be proceeded by various steps like intuition, interpretation, and integration [6]. The first two steps are proceeded by the individual researchers, whereas the third step of integration is a group process. The development of interpretation skills through integrated practices, understanding, adjusting, and compromising will lead to a newer path for learning [7]. When the process is clearly defined, it can be institutionalized by higher stakeholders.

8.4   The Need for Research Infrastructure

Global research stands still due to a lack of knowledge translation [8]. The process of knowledge transfer is dependent on the effort of stakeholders at different levels. The main disadvantage in implementing the knowledge transfer is the lack of knowledge management skills and adequate research infrastructure. The primary approach given by J. N. Lavis et al. [9] in 2006 was targeting the push, pull, and exchange efforts.

1. *The Push Approach:* This approach helps the researchers to disseminate the research findings outside the scientific community. Artificial intelligence can be used to scan all the available research literature of the faculty research, postgraduate dissertation, Ph.D. thesis, and other undergraduate research evidence of the organization. The research information can be easily disseminated to the general public and researchers.
2. *Pull Approach:* This approach targets the health system managers and policymakers to bridge the gap between the two ends; the researchers and the society that uses the research evidence. The pull approach is used to irrigate various research decision-making processes and to promote the use of research in decision-making. Self-assessment tools enhance the capacity to discover and utilize various research evidence in decision-making. This approach helps in training researchers and faculties to focus on research findings, creating research

evidence, and using it in clinical decision-making [9]. Creating an open-access system to exhibit all organization research to reach other scientific communities.
3. *The Exchange Approach:* It focuses on sustaining an active relation between the researcher, managing team and policy leaders. This approach targets the initiation of interactive research workshops and monitoring researches [9].

8.5   Research Infrastructure

Research infrastructure can be chiefly divided into four core areas: The resources, the faculties, the environment, and administration/organization.

The required resources can be further subcategorized as follows (Fig. 8.1):
(a) *Human resource:* Adequate samples or patients should be available. The organization should practice ethical guidelines of research. The hospitals indulged in clinical trials or other research studies should provide free investigation and excellent healthcare services to ensure the safety of the patients. Another aspect of human resources like trained technicians and skillful staff should be adequately recruited.
(b) *Information technology (IT):* The organization should provide different medical data models to collect information like name, geographical location, medical history, planned procedure, pharmacy prescriptions, and contact addresses of the patients. The hospital information must be interconnected and accessible to researchers after ethical clearance from the institutional ethics committee. The IT should provide the medical data models to be readily exported in various forms like portable document file, Microsoft excel format, R statistics language, IBM SPSS Syntax file, HL7 clinical document architecture, CSV (comma separated values), and database template (SQL).
(c) *Logistics:* The basic need for the researcher is adequate training programs to develop research skills. Regular ethical committee meetings and monitoring committee approval should be timely approved. Freehand in the use of laboratory utilities and other approvals for machinery/instrument utility is required.
(d) *Faculties:* Passable number of faculties interested in research should be recruited. As currently, all medical institutions are facings a crisis in medical faculties, and they are continuously inundated with clinical, teaching, and accreditation duties. Faculties should be trained to be a part of inter-institutional collaboration, multidisciplinary collaboration, and transdisciplinary collaboration.
(e) *Infrastructure:* Investment in healthcare infrastructure allows an organization to develop specialized research knowledge for evidence-based medical practice [10]. Well-equipped research laboratories, adequate space for research, sophisticated laboratories, hospital information systems, well-connected software, and easy access to patient care are the basis for a rich research environment.
(f) *Administrative leader:* Organization leaders should take steps to establish a Memorandum of understanding with other institutions and research

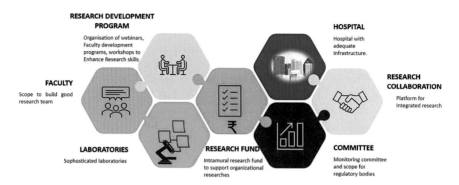

Fig. 8.1 Infrastructure for research

organizations. Policies and regulations to cater to the need of researchers should be initiated. Policies regarding the allotment of research funds for internal research faculties should be potentiated. Unbiased research environment for all cadre of the researcher. An incentivized approach will motivate the junior researcher to amplify the work effort.

(g) *National policies:* Regulations to strengthen ethics policies, to improve innovation and product development should be amplified. National level discussions to scale up a good laboratory and good clinical practices. Policies to build upon the health innovation system in technology development. Policies to amplify technology and knowledge transfer like (a) creating mechanisms for improvizing available technologies, (b) modes and methods for providing incentives and awards for international organizations that encourage knowledge transfer, (c) improvizing the development of piloting capacity in the public and private sector.

8.5.1 Common Challenges [11]

S. no.	Stakeholder	Challenges
1.	Healthcare system	Financial disincentives
2.	Healthcare organization	Lack of facilities, equipment, poor infrastructure
3.	Healthcare team	Local standards are not in par with desired practice
4.	Researcher	Attitude, knowledge, and skills
5.	Patients	Decrease adherence to drugs or devices
6.	Global changes	Constant changing health need
7.	Regulatory bodies	Mandatory research

8.6 Models to Assess the Impact of Implemented Research Infrastructure

The research supported by structures, skilled researchers, and technology to create quality research outcomes and sustain quality research can be assessed by recent assessment models. This model addresses the contribution of the underlying support infrastructure. Many funding organizations follow various models to evaluate the impact of research infrastructure on research outcomes. Research infrastructure is the basic need for a research project and the foundation for a long-term successful research system. The pipeline model used for programmatic research evaluation assesses the research outcome and the process. The model consists of input, process, output, outcomes, and impact. This traditional method analysis the research outcome by publication or citation metrics as these are easy to collect and quantitatively analyze. Whereas the actual analyses should focus quality of research faculties trained, the number of patients selected for research, and patients benefited [12].

In the current situation of evolution in research, many evaluative techniques have targeted qualitative analyses, newer exercises on "research excellence framework" and "accelerate framework" [13]. Many kinds of literature have shown the usage of various tailored pipeline models to evaluate a research infrastructure. In spite of multifaceted models and frameworks to substantiate the funding organization, the evaluation of research infrastructure is challenging. The newer models like the platform model have three platform analyses comprising Platform A, B, and C. Platform A analysis the research delivery system, and Platform B assesses the research sample and equipment. Platform C assesses the research facility, research workplace, and bio-resource. The platform model assesses the complete research infrastructure on all aspects of resources and facilities required to support research [14].

To avoid the pitfall of the two models, both the model can be fused, and a parallel framework can be developed using the pipeline model and platform framework [15]. To meet the demand of growing global health need the modern world research should reflect modern world evaluation. The evaluation models should be designed and implemented as per the organization's research needs. The stakeholders should design policies and regulations to evaluate the research infrastructure for high research outcomes.

8.6.1 Exhortations for Achieving High Yield Research

An advanced and high-quality research outcome can be achieved only by a multidimensional approach. A multifacet approach can provide a rich research atmosphere in an organization [15].

Advance training for faculties is the pillar for achieving high research outcomes. Workshops to improve research skills and gain knowledge of recent advances in health care. The research finding has to be adequately disseminated to the public and researchers by publications [16]. Conferences, seminars, workshops, and presentations are the other best means to bridge the knowledge lacunae. Creating a research network will help in data sharing among peer researchers and scale up collaborative research.

Policies to support the research environment in accord with legislation, regulations, and government policies as [17]
1. Collaborative research with other organizations and industries.
2. Faculty exchange program between hospitals, institutions, and industries.
3. Policies for advanced healthcare training and clinical practices.
4. Policies to benefit public health needs.

Improvement in Heath's knowledge and attitude [18]: Faculty development program to improve clinical skills. Activities to change health-risk behavior such as strategies and campaigns. Potentiating unbiased and better-targeted allocation of resources.

Evidence-based medicine: Improvizing quality of health care by analyzing patient feedback and taking adequate measures to meet the needs. Cost containment and providing effective health services will benefit local communities.

An organization leader should direct researchers into research contracts and increase income from industries. Plan modes to attract R & D investment from various funding organizations within the nation and overseas [19]. Yielding income from intellectual property and filing patent and piloting it in the right direction towards marketing [20]. This initiation will provide a high-end infrastructure for producing good research and high research outcome.

8.7   Conclusion

The need for a good quality research can be fulfilled by providing a platform to inculcate the researcher with adequate competencies. The ability for a researcher to conduct research depends not only on cognitive skills but also on communication skills, interpersonal skills, organizational skills, and personal motivation. A well-established infrastructure will provide support for long-term research and indirectly paves the path for evidence-based practice. Reforms in policies to support research environment will contribute to global healthcare system.

Case Scenario
A 54-year-female professor named Dr. Rahani who was working with a research organization has joined a medical institution. She wants to establish an infrastructure for high research outcomes. How can Dr. Rahani train her faculties to become good researchers? What are the various strategies she can adopt to evaluate the adequacy of research infrastructure at her institution?

References

1. Stefanadis CI. Characteristics of the good researcher: innate talent or acquired skills? Hellenic J Cardiol. 2006;47:52–3.
2. Rumman AAA, Alheet AF. The role of researcher competencies in delivering successful research. Inf Knowl Manag. 2019;9(1):29–32.
3. Cheruvelil KS, Soranno PA, Weathers KC, Hanson PC, Goring SJ, Filstrup CT, et al. Creating and maintaining high-performing collaborative research teams: the importance of diversity and interpersonal skills. Front Ecol Environ. 2014;12(1):31–8.
4. Willenberg KM. Attributes of successful leaders in research. Res Manag Rev. 2014;20(1):n1.
5. Shmatko NJF. Researchers' competencies in the coming decade: attitudes towards and expectations of the Russian innovation system. Foresight. 2016;18(3):340–54.
6. Lawrence TB, Mauws MK, Dyck B, Kleysen RF. The politics of organizational learning: integrating power into the 4I framework. Acad Manage Rev. 2005;30(1):180–91.
7. Crossan MM, Lane HW, White RE. An organizational learning framework: from intuition to institution. Acad Manage Rev. 1999;24(3):522–37.
8. Légaré F, Borduas F, MacLeod T, Sketris I, Campbell B, Jacques AJ. Partnerships for knowledge translation and exchange in the context of continuing professional development. J Contin Educ Health Prof. 2011;31(3):181–7.
9. Ellen ME, Lavis JN, Ouimet M, Grimshaw J, Bédard P-O. Determining research knowledge infrastructure for healthcare systems: a qualitative study. Implement Sci. 2011;6(1):1–5.
10. Ryu C, Kim YJ, Chaudhury A, Rao HR. Knowledge acquisition via three learning processes in enterprise information portals: learning-by-investment, learning-by-doing, and learning-from-others. Manag Inf Syst Q. 2005;29:245–78.
11. Grimshaw JM, Eccles MP, Walker AE, Thomas RE. Changing physicians' behavior: what works and thoughts on getting more things to work. J Contin Educ Health Prof. 2002;22(4): 237–43.
12. Grazier KL, Trochim WM, Dilts DM, Kirk R. Estimating return on investment in translational research: methods and protocols. Eval Health Prof. 2013;36(4):478–91.
13. De Giacomo O. Societal impact of research infrastructures final protocol. Accelerating Europe's leading research infrastructures. Brussels: European Commission; 2019.
14. Raftery J, Hanney S, Greenhalgh T, Glover M, Blatch-Jones A. Models and applications for measuring the impact of health research: update of a systematic review for the Health Technology Assessment programme. Health Technol Assess. 2016;20(76):1–254.
15. Zakaria S, Grant J, Luff J. Fundamental challenges in assessing the impact of research infrastructure. Health Res Policy Syst. 2021;19(1):1–9.
16. Kok MO, Schuit AJ. Contribution mapping: a method for mapping the contribution of research to enhance its impact. Health Res Policy Syst. 2012;10(1):1–16.
17. Cohen G, Schroeder J, Newson R, King L, Rychetnik L, Milat AJ, et al. Does health intervention research have real world policy and practice impacts: testing a new impact assessment tool. Health Res Policy Syst. 2015;13(1):1–12.
18. Graham KE, Chorzempa HL, Valentine PA, Magnan JJRE. Evaluating health research impact: development and implementation of the Alberta Innovates–Health Solutions impact framework. Res Eval. 2012;21(5):354–67.
19. Donovan C. The Australian Research Quality Framework: a live experiment in capturing the social, economic, environmental, and cultural returns of publicly funded research. New Dir Eval. 2008;2008(118):47–60.
20. Cruz Rivera S, Kyte DG, Aiyegbusi OL, Keeley TJ, Calvert MJ. Assessing the impact of healthcare research: a systematic review of methodological frameworks. PLoS Med. 2017;14 (8):e1002370.

Agreement and MOU: Ethical and Legal Aspects of Funding for Healthcare Research

9

A. R. Srinivasan

Ethics is knowing the difference between what you have a right to do and what is right to do

Potter Stewart

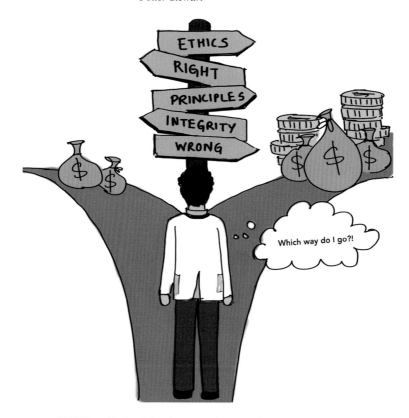

Agreement and MOU—ethical and legal aspects of funding for healthcare research

A. R. Srinivasan (✉)
Biochemistry Department, Mahatma Gandhi Medical College and Research Institute, Sri Balaji Vidyapeeth, Pondicherry, India

S. C. Parija, V. Kate (eds.), *Grant writing for medical and healthcare professionals*, https://doi.org/10.1007/978-981-19-7018-4_9

103

Objectives
- To appraise the reader of the distinguishing features between an agreement and an MoU vis-à-vis ethical and legal aspects of funding healthcare research.
- To prompt the reader towards a better understanding of funding opportunities for health research by projecting the essential ethical and legal aspects.
- To provide an insight into the health services research funding with reference to ethical and legal aspects.
- To inform the readers on the various alternative modalities with respect to MoUs and agreements.
- To provide the discerning reader an opportunity for comprehending a few appropriate case scenarios on the pertinent ethical and legal aspects of funded research in the realms of health care, followed by summary.

9.1   Introduction

In recent years, healthcare research has witnessed pronounced changes that have now become synonymous with research from the perspectives of a multidisciplinary approach. The approach is comprehensive and encompasses a wide gamut of facilities and opportunities that include organizational core structures, well-defined processes, discrete and focused technologies, and societal and psycho-social considerations. Special mention needs to be made of the attributes that govern access to quality health care, the desired quality and cost of health care, and holistic well-being. As far as the perspective frontiers of research in the realms of health care are concerned, it is the individuals, families, other stakeholders, organizations, nodal institutions, and communities that occupy the center stage. Hence, it is in the fitness of things that whenever the considerations of funding for health services (care) research are taken into due account, the aforementioned perspective frontiers of research should necessarily encompass ethical and legal aspects of funding. These need to be clearly delineated while effecting an agreement or MoU [1–4].

Moreover, it needs to be emphasized that the major ethical issues in facilitating the conduct of research in health care have to be essentially taken into account [5, 6]. They are (a) Obtaining Informed consent, (b) Principle of *Beneficence* (Do no harm) (c) Tenet governing *Respect for anonymity and upholding confidentiality* (d) *Respect for protecting privacy.*

The flow chart denoting the contents of this chapter is depicted in Fig. 9.1.

9.2   Health Services Research (HSR) Funding: Ethical and Legal Aspects

HSR is dynamic. Innovations in health policy acquire great relevance. Various issues governing medical insurance, claim, coverage, and factors hampering the utilization of care are pronouncedly conspicuous. The healthcare industry reflects a dynamic nature. In view of this inherent issue, HSR has a major role to play especially with

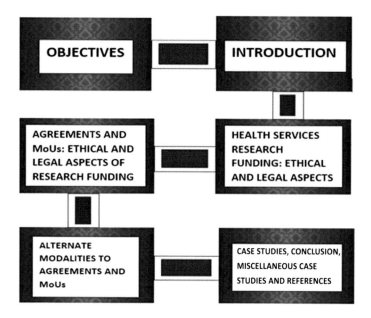

Fig. 9.1 Flowchart depicting the contents of the chapter titled agreement and MoU—ethical and legal aspects of funding for healthcare research

respect to the impact that it affects patient outcomes as related to safety, cost, and comfort [7].

As per the documented literature, the Nuremberg Code of 1947 denotes the earliest global document on the ethics of research involving human subjects/volunteers. This document lays vivid emphasis on the facets related to providing voluntary consent. It needs to be highlighted that in the year 1964, the World Medical Association came up with the bedrock guidelines for enabling research on humans (Declaration of Helsinki). Since then, several revisions have been effected. As a significant development, the Belmont Report was released in the United States that emphatically underlined the three rudimentary ethical principles for research involving human subjects, namely respect for persons, acknowledgment, and justice. The Belmont report emerged in the year 1979. All of these principles underlined therein play a pivotal role with respect to the wide gamut of ethical and legal aspects of funding in healthcare research [8–10].

In the year 2017, the comprehensive National Ethical Guidelines for the conduct of *Biomedical and Health Research* involving human participants was formulated by the apex council of India, namely the Indian Council of Medical Research, New Delhi. These guidelines depict *hitherto* less visited areas in ethical research, including public health research, behavioral sciences, disaster management, biological materials, biobanking, and vulnerable populations [11].

Clinical research tests new therapeutic modalities on volunteers. Whereas the eventual goal of clinical research is to upgrade the existing clinical knowledge and improve patient care, all relevant aspects signifying ethics and legal validity acquire mandatory consideration. In order that the conclusions emanating from clinical research to be valid and applicable, the research must be conducted intentionally through systematic interventions and subsequent data collection and analysis. Sponsors should take cognizance of all of these facts while sanctioning extramural research grants that should culminate in legally valid and ethically intact study results for the larger benefit of the community [12].

9.3 MoUs, Agreements

MoUs and Agreements denote integral parts of transacting business in any establishment, be it public or private. Quite frequently, these two terms, namely MoU and Agreement are used interchangeably and inadvertently. As a matter of fact, it is imperative to comprehend the differences. Once adept at the distinction between these two terms, the reader would get easily acquainted with the alternative modalities to the same (Agreements, MoUs). However, the fact remains that the ethical and legal aspects of funding healthcare research need to be vividly portrayed in such documents.

The distinguishing features of an Agreement/Contract and MoU are portrayed in Fig. 9.2 and Table 9.1.

9.4 Types of Agreements in Biomedical Research (Alternate Modalities to Agreements and MoUs)

There are several types of agreements that are in vogue, as related to biomedical research. These are highlighted below (see also Fig. 9.3) [13, 14].

1. **Allocation of Rights** document is basically defined as a non-monetary agreement that establishes the rights between parties to the existing endeavors and also those that would be taken up in the future, in the realms of intellectual property.

Fig. 9.2 The distinguishing features of an agreement and MoU

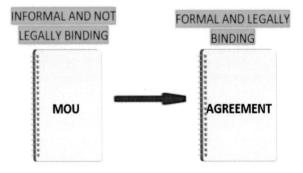

Table 9.1 Essential differences between an informal MOU and a formal agreement/contract

Context and relevance	MOU	Agreement (contract)
Definition	Document to depict that the parties have embarked on achieving a common objective	Document to depict that two or more parties have consented to dwell on a legally binding agreement
Enforceability	Not legally enforceable	Legally enforceable
Overall aim	The parties have a mutual understanding in a written form	The obligation of the parties taken into account Risk mitigation in place
Content specificity	Subject matter spelled out Objectives and purpose enumerated Essential terms available as a summary	Essentially refers to a proposal by one party and acceptance by the other
Financial consideration	No exchange of money	Money exchange is mandatory
Most optimal utility	Profit is not the main purpose of the relationship	Profit is the main purpose of the relationship
Resolution of disputes that may arise	Resolution through mutual discussions and dialog	Arbitration or litigation essential

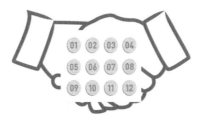

Fig. 9.3 Alternate modalities to Agreements and MoUs (Twelve modalities for Biomedical Research) 1. Allocation of Rights, 2. Collaborative Research Agreement, 3. Consortium Agreement, 4. Data Use Agreement, 5. Interagency Cooperation Contract, 6. Material Transfer Agreements, 7. Memorandum of Understanding, 8. Non-Disclosure Agreement, 9. Service agreements, 10. Sponsored Research Agreement, 11. Subaward, 12. Teaming Agreement

2. **Collaborative Research Agreements** are aptly regarded as contracts effected between the host institute and one or more organizations that would endeavor together in the conduct of a research program. These automatically call for ethical and legal aspects of funding.
3. **Consortium Agreement** is described as a contract that would afford multiple sponsors to participate in group endeavors in supporting research. In such a case, the outcomes of the research would be shared equally. Greater implications of ethics and legal validity are felt here that are mainly attributed to the presence of multiple sponsors.

4. **Data Use Agreement** is a non-funded agreement that is executed between two parties where either one or both parties exchange data securely. In such a scenario, research data and publications are shared in accordance with the existing policies of the higher education institutions and statutory bodies/ governments. In addition, the guidelines stipulated for healthcare institutions also need to be essentially followed.
5. **Interagency Cooperation Contract** frequently refers to a written agreement between the agencies of a state under which the goods or services are provided. The office of the sponsored projects holds the key. Research concerning pharmaceutical products is relevant in this context.
6. **Material Transfer Agreements** are contract-based documents utilized for the purpose of procuring various biological and research materials developed by non-profit organizations, public, and private sectors/industries.
7. **Memorandum of Understanding** (MoU) is termed a contract between two or more parties joining hands to create a research or academic partnership. However, the MOU is not a legally binding agreement and hence should not essentially address formal plans including those meant for compensation, licensing rights, etc.
8. **Non-disclosure Agreement** or a proprietary information agreement is a legal contract between a minimum of two parties that point towards confidential matters that could be shared with one another for certain well-defined and specific purposes sans generalized use.
9. **Service agreements** denote legally binding contracts. These are oriented towards the sale of goods/services from the higher education/research institution to another entity. These agreements encompass terms and conditions relevant to the work of chosen interest.
10. **Sponsored Research Agreement** is effected when an external organization/ institution/industry provides funding to a higher education/research organization in order to support an earmarked research project with an expectation of receiving certain deliverables.
11. **Subaward** is nothing but an agreement with a third-party organization executing a small, but a well-defined portion of a funded research project. The terms of the subcontract are governed by the prime agreement. It is imperative that all the subcontracts be monitored to ensure that there is complete compliance with the laid down rules of the subcontract.
12. **Teaming Agreement** is synonymous with a binding agreement between one or more organizations that are endeavoring on cooperative research with reference to a prime sponsor. The lead proposing organization is usually a governmental organization.

Having said that, it needs to be emphasized that Agreements and MoUs are frequently encountered in healthcare research, and hence the ethical and legal aspects of funding are considered significant largely in the light of the two, namely Agreements and MoUs.

9.5 The Distinction Between Agreements and MoUs

The essential facts regarding Agreements have been clearly delineated in the Indian Contract Act, 1872 (refer to Section 10). This act clearly states what agreements are about. An agreement essentially portrays content for the purpose of binding each other with the terms of the agreement. It needs to be emphasized that upon violation of the terms of the proposed agreement, the other party would go for legal redressal. Hence, it needs to be reiterated that an agreement is most appropriately regarded as a legal document that is essentially formed following the finalization of the intended mutual benefits, and it is synonymous with the binding document. Hence, in sponsored research, there is greater accountability with respect to the ethics and legality of the endeavor (Table 9.1).

With reference to an MoU, we need to take cognizance of the fact that both the parties had announced their intent, besides exuding commitment to faithfully follow the intention in future endeavors. However, no valid contract manifests in an MoU. In the event of a party committing an act that reflects on the reliance and validity of the *MoU* under consideration and also sustains any loss in the process, we can make amends without enforcing the *same*. In general, an MoU specifies mutually accepted expectations between the parties, as related to common objective(s). In a few instances such as those observed in the United States, an MoU is considered equivalent to a Letter of Intent which is merely a non-binding written agreement.

9.6 Points to be Remembered While Drafting an Agreement or MoU: from the Viewpoint of Funding Research

Though, in general, an MoU is not legally binding, the inclusion of a provision with the intention of making it legally viable could be in place with implications related to confidentiality, privacy, or resolution to overcome disputes, etc. Under these defined considerations, the MoU could become legally binding.

It is the ethical aspect of research in general that calls for the use of mild and suave language which does not necessarily cast strict obligations or restrictions upon the parties at the time of drafting an MOU. Inclusion of immoderate details with regard to payment, promptness of services, etc. should be eschewed [15].

9.7 Reflection on the Ethical and Legal Aspects of Funding Healthcare Research in the Drafting of MoUs and Agreements

Prior to drafting an MoU or agreement, we need to know the various components of the same and with particular reference to the ethical and legal aspects of funding research.

1. *Title:* The descriptive name of the MoU/Agreement should necessarily reflect the nature of the intended transactions between the parties spelled out in non-controversial, clear, and euphemistic terms.
2. *Identification of the Parties:* This should clearly delineate the reciprocal desire of both the parties signifying equal commitment in the joint endeavor. Conflicts with any existing MoU or agreement entered by the organization between or among the parties *including* the third party must necessarily be avoided. Since this document is in accordance with an established convention, it should necessarily be elaborated with the assistance/on the advice of the legal personnel.
3. *Background:* This section should contain non-controversial gist of the proposed endeavor in the light of the existing scenario. The background should also reveal important facets of the ethical and legal aspects of funding research.
4. *Legal and ethical validity:* The MoU/Agreement should contain the substance that is legally binding as well as retains the relevance to any rule defining appropriate procedures to which the parties are subjected, both in terms of legal and ethical validity.
5. *Purpose:* Should be clearly explained in unambiguous terms.
6. *Consideration of an Agreement:* This should reflect ethically driven mutual promises that may or may not be legally binding, depending upon the fact as to whether it is an Agreement or MoU.
   If it is an international agreement, the implications of foreign exchange have to be underlined emphatically.
7. *Joint Undertaking and Responsibilities*:
8. *Indemnification Clause:* (1) Compensatory damages are frequently encountered that warrant the disbursement of cash to necessarily reimburse for costs in order to compensate for the specified loss and (2) Consequential and incidental damages meant for confronting losses caused by the breach that was originally deemed imminent are mentioned herein. Other important clauses including termination and arbitration are also rendered feasible as admissible under the existing rules and regulations.
   It must however be clearly imbibed that every contract or agreement should be carefully developed with comprehensive insight and focused introspection into the minds of parties. The clauses may be regarded as standard. However, the relevant facts might vary with the nature and type of the party, as deemed mutually appropriate.

9.8   The Ethical and Legal Aspects of Funding Research in Health Care

The following points are to be taken into strict consideration while granting funds to the researchers in health care. These points acquire relevance with respect to both the ethical and legal aspects of funding in healthcare research, as revealed in the Agreements/MoUs.

1. Patient safety 2. Effectiveness 3. Timeliness 4. Patient-centric 5. Efficiency 6. Equity.

The various aspects related to the crux of the ethical and legal considerations concerning the conduct of clinical research acquire relevance since it involves human participants. These facets draw the attention of policymakers, attorneys, clinical researchers, and other stakeholders.

Legal and ethical issues form an integral component of contemporary research, as related to the subject and researcher [16]. Researchers should be conversant with the major international guidelines and regional, national, and international differences in legislation. Hence, specific ethical advice should be sought at the level of individual Ethics Review Committees. One must take due note of the fact that the required financial support for research is drawn from several sources. It is the inherent responsibility of the researchers that the funds and resources allocated for the specific purpose of carrying out research in health care are utilized properly. Utilization of funds without any misappropriation or misconduct is a prerogative of the researchers.

The Institute Human Ethics Committee plays a nodal role in the proper utilization of funds. The role played by the funding agency in ensuring the proper utilization of funds cannot be underestimated. It is imperative that well-defined principles and codes are in place for ensuring the proper utilization of these funds. The basic requirements to conduct any type of research include truthfulness, sustained interest, and motivation. These ingredients are facilitated by academic, administrative, peer, and financial support.

Several sources are presently available for carrying out quality evidence-based research and include intramural and extramural grants. The extramural grants could be obtained from government organizations, international organizations of repute, corporate sectors, and non-government organizations including philanthropic individuals and groups.

Researchers have a huge moral responsibility in ensuring that the resources are optimally utilized without any semblance of misconduct. It is in this regard that the respective institute ethics committees, in association with the funding organizations should take due cognizance of the fact and act in a manner befitting the ethos.

The host institutes should necessarily patronize policies and protocols, including those that directly and indirectly govern research promotion. Utmost care has to be exercised in promulgating ethically and legally intact endeavors which will lay down the tenets of accountable research practice, besides clearly identifying the responsibilities of the host institutions and their avid researchers in diverse areas including data management, authorship, conflict of interest/competing interest, supervision of mentees and research trainees, and most significantly the handling of funds fostered by an ethically intact approach. Mention must be made of the fact that the Missenden code was primarily developed to address the variegated issues and challenges posed by the funding sources in a robust and transparent manner.

The host institutes fostering research need to establish ethics committees mandatorily in order to monitor the sources of funding. Furthermore, the ethics committees need to ensure that the research funding is acknowledged in all publications. The

Indian Council of Medical Research (ICMR) emphatically recommends these attributes.

So long as the bonafide intention of the organization is vivid, the scenario is deemed appropriate. Furthermore, if the ethical, as well as the legal aspects of healthcare research funding, are duly taken care of, we would escape from the threat of ambiguity or bias. As a matter of fact, no research whatsoever is truly independent. This is because of the fact that funding has to essentially happen. Utmost importance needs to be accorded to the credence of the research endeavor in the process. It is also imperative that we need to be transparent about the funding and resources that had largely contributed to their research, besides focusing on possible quality publications of high impact and also intellectual property endeavors including copyrights, patents, and technology transfer.

9.9 The Basic Structure of Ethical Consideration of Funding for Research in Health Care

It is the prerogative of the institutes to keep themselves abreast of the framework that would tell them as to whether they should accept external funding for the purpose of carrying out academic, research, or other endeavors. The matter and responsibility rest with the individual in identifying whether there are any sensitive ethical and legal issues and if so, ways and means to mitigate the same. The investigator (s) should be careful in accepting the grants from the sources, especially under dubious circumstances that would either cast aspersions or bring disrepute. Circumstances citing the precarious position, wherein the funder could use the results of the study for depicting unethical practices need to be avoided at any cost.

9.10 Case Studies with Reference to Ethical and Legal Aspects of Funded Research [15–17]

Case Study 1
Situation: Clinical trial in Oncology.
Nature of the Clinical trial: Randomized, single-blinded, placebo-controlled study of a drug D that might prove beneficial to the patient P.
Duration of the Clinical Trial: One-year.
Evaluation at the end of the first half of the study period: No signs of improvement for the patient. In fact, deterioration in general health was perceptible.
Observations by the Principal investigator (PI) at the end of the first half of the study period: The PI obtained reports concerning the progress of the research subjects enrolled in both the arms, namely therapeutic and placebo. A preliminary report pointed to the beneficial effect of the chemotherapeutic drug.
Patient-PI discussion: During the routine follow-up, the patient asked the PI if he/she is in the treatment arm or the placebo arm. The PI was well aware that the patient was in the placebo arm. The patient requested that if he was in the placebo

arm be switched over to the treatment arm in order to reap the projected benefits of the novel therapeutic modality.

Case Study 2
Situation: National HIV trial was halted owing to issues related to patient rights.

Nature and duration of the clinical trial: A major study (1 year) funded by the Government to determine whether the anti-viral drug AV would prove to be an effective, preventative therapeutic modality against the HIV.

Progress of the Clinical trial: Halted owing to protests regarding the terms of the trial. The trial was supposed to have enrolled N number of patients. "Women who became infected during the trial would not be offered treatment. Instead, they would be referred to nearby healthcare services." This was not tenable, as it had both ethical and legal issues that were not conforming to the established principles of funded healthcare research.

9.11 Ethical and Legal Considerations in Funded Research, with Reference to the Above-Cited Case Studies

Four major considerations have evolved from the case studies
1. The double hat predicament.
2. Ethics involved in the process of randomization and blinding.
3. Ethical and legal issues concerning preliminary data.
4. Ethical use of placebo.

- The first and foremost obligation of the physician (PI) is towards the patient concern, safety, and comfort. However, as the PI in a clinical trial, he/she has a competing obligation towards other essential facets including recruitment and retention of patients.
- The investigator or the PI has to perform non-therapeutic procedures including randomization, blinding and administration of the drug, adherence to stringent protocol, etc. that do not directly serve patients and instead might even place them in jeopardy (Double hat predicament).
- Helsinki Declaration, Brazil 2013 Para 4: **It is the inherent duty of the physician to promote and safeguard the health of patients, including those who are involved in medical research. The physician's knowledge and conscience are dedicated to the fulfillment of this duty.**
- Para 3 **"The health of my patient will be my first consideration..." "A physician shall act in the patient's best interest when providing medical care."**
- Helsinki Declaration, Brazil 2013 Para 14 **The physician may combine medical research with medical care only to the extent that the research is justified by its potential preventive, diagnostic, or therapeutic value and if the physician**

**has good reason to believe that participation in the research study will not
adversely affect the health of the patients who serve as research subjects.**

9.12   Conclusion

To conclude, Agreements/Contracts and MOUs are typified by the presence of
distinct features. While drafting an agreement or MOU in the realms of healthcare
research, care must be taken to uphold patient safety, comfort, and satisfaction.
Further, organizational ethics holds the key to patient-related endeavors in funded
research. The relational ethics depicting patients and related stakeholders is cardinal
in funded research. Legal aspects and issues are ingrained in funded research and
need to be comprehended by the parties, prior to the process of formalization
(Fig. 9.4).

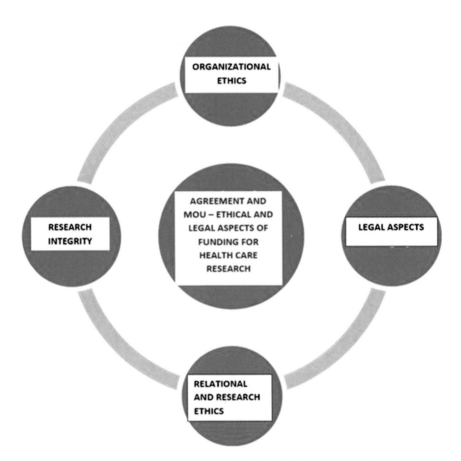

Fig. 9.4 Summary of ethical and legal aspects of funding for healthcare research

Case Scenario 1
Mr. X was recruited following informed consent to participate in a clinical trial that had featured an anti-cancer drug. The Principal Investigator (PI) of the Clinical Trial was Dr. Y. Mr. X had malignancy and was already on treatment as per the established, conventional, rational protocol underlined for the treatment of cancer. The clinical trial essentially centered around a randomized, single-blinded, placebo-controlled investigation of a newly developed drug that might confer benefits on the patient with the type and nature of cancer that Mr. X was afflicted with. Furthermore, the clinical trial was planned for a total period of 1 year. At the culmination of the stipulated period of 1 year, first hand and genuine data was made available that could serve as an objective indicator of the efficacy of the therapeutic modality. Midway through the study, Mr. X's general condition had deteriorated. Dr. Y was continuously apprised of the progress of the study and categorically understood that the drug had beneficial effects. In the meantime, Mr. X had made a plea that if he is in the placebo arm, the PI Dr. Y might use his good offices to switch over the former (Mr. X) from the placebo to the therapeutic arm of the drug trial. If done so, Mr. X expressed his desire that he can then receive the possible benefits of the new treatment.

1. Comment on the predicament faced by Dr. Y with particular reference to the ethical aspects of funded research.
2. What are the ethical issues that ought to be necessarily taken into consideration in funded research?
3. Comment on the common ethical issues in clinical trials.
4. It is ethically not permitted to conduct placebo controlled trials in the event of the availability of a proven therapeutic modality for the clinical condition under focus.

Case Scenario 2
21,687 subjects were enrolled into the study that pointed to a randomized trial. All the enrolled subjects had an episode of Acute Myocardial Infarction (AMI). The study groups were randomized to streptokinase or placebo. Primary endpoint which essentially denotes whether the new modality is better at preventing AMI-related mortality in comparison to the standard therapy accounted for the following statistics at the end of 150 days: Streptokinase 8.8% as against Placebo 14%.

1. Comment on the ethical implications of the above-mentioned trial with reference to placebo-based trials in highly morbid conditions.
2. When streptokinase is regarded as the gold standard for treating AMI, is it acceptable to call for a clinical trial by including a placebo group.
3. Considering the fact that any clinical trial is planned with a view to generating authentic data for future endeavors mainly aimed at efficacy and safety of the therapeutic modality under investigation, is it alright to sacrifice the safety and lives of the subjects included in the present clinical trial.

4. Comment on the compensation package with reference to the above-mentioned clinical trial.

References

1. Srinivasan K, Fredrick J, Gupta R, Singh N. Funding opportunities for health research in India—a technical scan. Indian J Public Health. 2020;64(4):421–4. https://doi.org/10.4103/ijph.IJPH_9_20.
2. Dako-Gyeke P, Asampong E, Afari E, Launois P, Ackumey M, Opoku-Mensah K, Dery S, Akweongo P, Nonvignon J, Aikins M. Capacity building for implementation research: a methodology for advancing health research and practice. Health Res Policy Syst. 2020;18(1): 53. https://doi.org/10.1186/s12961-020-00568-y.
3. Cartier Y, Creatore MI, Hoffman SJ, Potvin L. Priority-setting in public health research funding organisations: an exploratory qualitative study among five high-profile funders. Health Res Policy Syst. 2018;16(1):53. https://doi.org/10.1186/s12961-018-0335-8.
4. van der Graaf P, Blank L, Holding E, Goyder E. What makes a 'successful' collaborative research project between public health practitioners and academics? A mixed-method review of funding applications submitted to a local intervention evaluation scheme. Health Res Policy Syst. 2021;19(1):9. https://doi.org/10.1186/s12961-020-00671-0.
5. Bhutta ZA. Ethics in international health research: a perspective from the developing world. Bull World Health Organ. 2002;80(2):114–20.
6. Frith L. Why health services research needs bioethics. J Med Ethics. 2017;43(10):655–6. https://doi.org/10.1136/medethics-2017-104247.
7. Liaw ST, Tam CW. Research ethics and approval process: a guide for new GP researchers. Aust Fam Physician. 2015;44(6):419–22.
8. Bosch-Capblanch X, Abba K, Prictor M, Garner P. Contracts between patients and healthcare practitioners for improving patients' adherence to treatment, prevention and health promotion activities. Cochrane Database Syst Rev. 2007;2007(2):CD004808. https://doi.org/10.1002/14651858.CD004808.pub3.
9. Lorente R, Antonanzas F, Rodriguez-Ibeas R. Implementation of risk-sharing contracts as perceived by Spanish hospital pharmacists. Health Econ Rev. 2019;9:25. https://doi.org/10.1186/s13561-019-0242-x.
10. Mandal J, Parija M, Parija SC. Ethics of funding of research. Trop Parasitol. 2012;2(2):89–90. https://doi.org/10.4103/2229-5070.105172.
11. Mathur R, Swaminathan S. National Ethical Guidelines for Biomedical and Health Research involving human participants, 2017: a commentary. Indian J Med Ethics. 2018;3(3):201–4. https://doi.org/10.20529/IJME11.2018.065.
12. Parks MR, Disis ML. Conflicts of interest in translational research. J Transl Med. 2004;2(1):28. https://doi.org/10.1186/1479-5876-2-28.
13. Chopra SS. Industry funding of clinical trials: benefit or bias? JAMA. 2003;290:113.
14. Johns MEE, Barnes M, Florencio PS. Restoring balance to industry–academia relationships in an era of institutional financial conflicts of interest. JAMA. 2003;289(6):741–6.
15. Bekelman JE, Yan LI, Gross CP. Scope and impact of financial conflicts of interest in biomedical research. JAMA. 2003;289(4):454–65.
16. Bonham VH. Chapter 12—Legal issues in clinical research. In: Gallin JI, Ognibene FP, Johnson LL, editors. Principles and practice of clinical research. 4th ed. New York: Academic Press; 2018. p. 161–75. https://doi.org/10.1016/B978-0-12-849905-4.00012-5.
17. https://www.crc.gov.my/wpcontent/uploads/documents/intranet/GCP/05_Final_Edited_Ethics_Ethical_problems_in_clinical_trial.pdf.

Writing an Impressive Cover Page (Covering Letter) and Abstract for Grant Proposal Application

Nirmal Kumar Ganguly and Gautam Kumar Saha

Creativity is seeing what others see & thinking what no one else ever thought

Albert Einstein

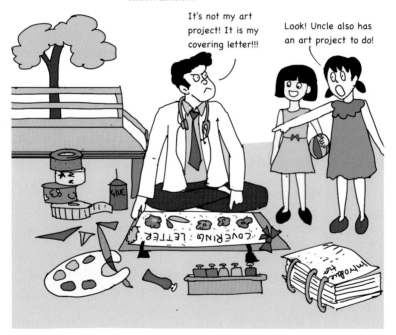

Writing an impressive cover page

N. K. Ganguly (✉)
Former Director General, Indian Council of Medical Research, New Delhi, India

Apollo Hospitals Educational and Research Foundation (AHERF), New Delhi, India

G. K. Saha
Apollo Hospitals Educational and Research Foundation (AHERF), New Delhi, India

S. C. Parija, V. Kate (eds.), *Grant writing for medical and healthcare professionals*,
https://doi.org/10.1007/978-981-19-7018-4_10

Objectives
- Understand the basic principles of writing a cover letter and abstract
- Realise the various mistakes to avoid when writing a cover letter and abstract

10.1   Introduction: The Need for Cover Letter and Abstract

The basis of any relationship is communication which conveys trust. Gaining financial commitment from scientific grant agencies for new novel scientific projects requires gaining the trust and interest of the reviewers. Building a robust scientific proposal can ensure the grant agencies' commitment. Here the cover letter and abstract also play a vital role.

There is a marked difference between the abstract and executive summary. The proposal's critical points are mentioned concisely in the abstract. In comparison, the executive summary discusses in detail the significant points of the project venture. The critical point is that a cover letter comes at the beginning of the grant proposal. We tend to focus on first writing proposals, which is an important task. However, the cover letter has a greater significance as it introduces the grant writer, his ideas, and his organisation to the grant agency.

Abstract provides a view of the project proposal, conveying to the grant agency that the project's overall goals are similar to the grant agency's program.

10.2   How to Compose a Cover Letter for a Grant Proposal?

10.2.1 Salient Features of Cover Letter

Cover letters serve as an introduction to complete grant requests. A cover letter for a grant proposal letter should be no more than a single page long. We typically start to write it as if a synopsis of a book or thesis.

A cover letter can be considered the key that opens the doors to the grant agency. Hence, a cover letter's significance is paramount as a significant component of the grant application.

10.2.2 Make Grant Proposal the Soul of Cover Letter

Yes, the Grant proposal is the soul and backbone of the cover letter. So before starting to write the cover letter, ensure to understand the project's facts. To capture the interest of the reviewers, consider using a narrative structure in the cover letter.

Although the cover letter of a grant application may not be the most intriguing section, it is still a necessary item to secure financing. A cover letter is the first contact point for potential collaboration between the applicant's organisation and sponsors about a non-profit or profitable initiative although most likely, drafting a grant cover letter is the last activity of an applicant.

10.2.3 Cover Letter Needs Due Attention: Not A Simple Exercise

A letter might appear as a simple exercise, but one should carefully watch the progress at each step as letter will first step to convey the idea. One can correlate the letter to an office interview or going out for the first time meeting with a new friend, potential collaborator, or business partner. Although an interview or meeting, one's looks are not that important, however, one will have no excuse who does not work on oneself to have a presentable appearance; otherwise, then, things may become difficult.

Hence likewise, creating an excellent grant application cover letter is critical since it aids in capturing the attention of recipient grant agency officials. A crucial point that has to be emphasised repeatedly as a cover letter must stand out for grant agency program officers, as they may get hundreds of bids from various organisations. The following detail has to be a part of the cover letter [1]. Here are some pointers to help draft a successful grant proposal cover letter along with important aspects (Table 10.1).

10.2.3.1 Here is How to Compose A Cover Letter

The most important thing to remember when writing a "Grant application" is "Cover Letter", which shall be at the beginning. A grant application's average cover letter form should be no more than one page long. Make it an integral part of Grant's writing.

A thorough grant proposal's backbone is the cover letter. Consider it a synopsis of a book. Before proceeding to the first paragraph, one must begin a letter addressing the concerned person, including the contact's name, title, address, and other pertinent information. Here are a few things mentioned that although we think we know one has to be careful when writing the same.

- Double-check that the contact information is correct, even if it appears apparent. There are several examples of hastily written letters. No one wants their project halted due to a misspelling of the CEO or Director's name. Carry out fact-finding about grant agencies before writing a cover letter.
- One quickly finds the information one requires through a simple phone call, email, or just browsing up information on the Internet.
- Always, at the beginning sentence with "Dear" and then add unique titles like "Mister" or "Mrs" or academic titles like Prof. and Dr., or other appropriate salutation. A grant letter is to be treated as a personal letter of introduction to a person though the format may be formal.

10.2.3.2 Framing the Cover Letter to Seek Attention of Reader

Framing a cover letter is of vital importance. If this does not seem significant, the one who writes the letter is not focused on the task. One should consider it from the perspective of the grant agency's director or program officers who will do the reading. Leaders tend to be indolent. Read the cover letter to move forward, read from the first to last lines sensibly with care, and remove errors.

Table 10.1 The cover letter should include the following important aspects: this is explained in detail below

1	*Name and Address Receiver and Recipient*	At the top of your grant cover letter, use a formal title. A formal title is preferred by most professionals. This section can be in the header and the footer might include things like contact information. Another key consideration is the date on which the letter was sent. Contact information for the recipient is most essential especially when you are sending hard copies of the proposal and grant letter. It will be easy for receivers to contact you and provide an offer date if you provide these elements. It may also help you connect with your firm, particularly if you're preparing a proposal on your letterhead
2	*An overview of the organisation*	Include an introduction to your institute/university/company at the start of your grant application in the cover letter. This will assist peer reviewers to get a better understanding of your organization and its aims. Specific points about the organisation and mandate may be discussed in this section. The format can be set as follows: • This is the organisation's name • Values and purpose of the organisation • How long has your company been in existence? When writing this part, keep in mind that the entire letter's goal is to raise funds for your project initiative from your organisation, not the organisation itself. As a result, this data may be condensed to allow for greater discussion on the project itself
3	*A. Talk about the project's goal*	The aim of the project should be discussed in the body of the cover letter also. This is critical because it provides the grant auditor with a broad overview of your organisation's objectives are in synchrony with their agency mandate. You may share the web link of your institute for auditors to verify your profile and your organisation credentials
3.	*B. Project's prospects*	Depending on the novelty and type of the project you're working on, you may include as much information as you need to ensure that reviewers can understand the significance of the project completely even in brief. In the most successful cover letter, this information is frequently explained
4.	Describe why you're looking for money	The reviewers can explain why they require financing after they have a broad idea of the organisation and the project they are attempting to undertake. The following information should be highlighted: How do you intend to use funds? The sum of money that you're seeking for Why does your company require help? Another piece of information that may be included in this part is the reason why your organisation sought funds from the letter's recipient. However, if you're looking for money from a company or a person, this may be true
5	Emphasise the financial implications	In your grant letter, be sure you emphasise the importance of prospective financing. This is because it can assist peer reviewers to see how their suggestions can enhance your case directly. The following are some specific elements that should

(continued)

Table 10.1 (continued)

		be highlighted: Who can benefit from the project's benefits who can benefit from the project's benefits This information may persuade funders to support a project if they believe their contributions will have a beneficial impact on persons affected by the problem the organisation is attempting to tackle
6	Finish with a formal declaration	Experts frequently include a formal closing remark to the grant submission at the end of a successful cover letter. To the formal ending statement, here are a few things to add (next point)
7	Overview of the project	What can the project provide you? Thank you to the reviewers for considering your idea Closing sentences are usually two or three sentences long

Here are some helpful guidelines to follow when writing your cover letter for your grant application
The few unique points that need to be taken care of and are as follows

Give direct attention to the most critical aspects of the Grant Application, i.e. Cover Letter. Initial information in the cover letter reassures grant agencies that the applicant and his organisation are genuine contenders and that the application should be read and reviewed. The applicant cannot have an excuse if the information is missing or incorrect. Revise thoroughly so that no wrong information is in the cover letter or application. The applicant and the organisation will not be potential awardees of grants from the donor organisation in case of incomplete or wrong information. Everyone knows why we are drafting a cover letter for a grant application. It is right there in the title and the subject, the objective of the application. So the implication is that there is no need to stray from the topic and apologise.

10.2.4 Key Information and Features of Cover Letter

Using the steps mentioned in this section, one should be able to write grant applications of any size. A direct approach must be in the cover letter to state an organisation's initiatives on the most critical challenges. Explain why the organisation or foundation requires the grant and the mission and, most crucially, mention the requested budget. If the organisation applying for the grant involves a community initiative or a philanthropic group, its achievement will be there in the letter. In any case, keep it brief.

Keep the budget modest with rationale but never insufficient if it has the potential to
- Attract more significant funds, so it should be mentioned. It may be necessary sometimes to mention the budget if the grant agency's cover letter format requires it outright.

Table 10.2 Sample how cite in numbers the organisation achievements

• The organisation's four main goals are...
• The project will evolve through five phases...
• The authors have already published seven related studies......
• The organisation has conducted over 200 projects.....
• The investigators and the organisation have been awarded 20 research grants on average every 3 years for last 2 decades

- After introductory information in the following paragraph of the cover letter, must mention expenditure of modalities utilisation of the budget sought by the grant agency.
- Methods, strategies, and solutions for the project should be highlighted. The outright mention of the budget justification successfully communicates to the grant agencies with a strategy.
- The letter's structure is to communicate goals and strategies.
- Depending on the format, it may also contain graphic model files for visual presentation. Some authors prefer to use numbered samples for presenting achievement stats (Table 10.2).
- Initial concept validation information is sometimes essential to the funding agencies. When more considerable funding is required, a worthy endeavour is to test the concept through research. Suppose one had already carried out a pilot project and obtained initial results that need to be mentioned in the cover letter. The statement should be emphatic if the pilot project is successful. Also, suppose the organisation has carried out several other research projects similar to the one proposed in the grant application and has obtained extramural grants. In that case, that is a plus point that should be mentioned in the letter.
- Check and seek opinion: Make a cover sample letter and share it with friends and co-workers if one is unsure how to style a paragraph. As well as ask associates to write a paragraph that should be in sync with the grant application form. The applicant and their team have to read the preamble to the grant application and satisfy the questions asked informal application form. The colleague's main opinion should be if the cover letter is aligned and highlights project objectives aligned with the grant agency.

10.2.5 Main Highlights of Cover Letter

When there is hard evidence to defend an organisation's existing capability and reputation, few individuals can find a way to dispute it. In most cases, an organisation wants to back up each achievement with a certain number associated with it, like several grants awarded and the number of grants obtained, along with more facts. The outline is excellent, but simply putting a few numbers in a letter is insufficient. The strength of investigators and organisations needs to come out clearly yet in a concise way. Strive for a balance of simplicity and complexity [2].

The numbering provides a good structure, and the added information should make the writing appear more professional. Another excellent addition is providing a timeline with milestones and completion dates. Applicants can use the short bullet format for this. Project targets with timelines may be elaborate, but outline information can be written to signify the venture's feasibility. Timestamps might be months or quarters, depending on the project's length. In the last two sentences describing the organisation/institute/university structure is necessary. Describe the organisation's structure and relevant details, including the date of inception.

Remember, an applicant must write the grant application in great detail, along with the cover letter, which shall be reviewed and read by reviewers. Defining the applicant's approach and talents in the cover letter is unnecessary, but if the applicant can adequately explain concisely and fit it on one page, they can do so. However, the "Cover Letter" should also convey the idea of the mission as it will pave the way for the project to be shortlisted.

The cover letter should have all the information the grant agency will utilise to decide on a shortlisting project for further detailed review. The letter content should be read in a short time and should swiftly cover the facts regarding the organisation and structure after having explained the contents of the project proposed and its novelty mission in the first few sentences. One who is writing an application must highlight significant outcomes of the mission with a proposed budget for executing the plan is necessary. The mention of the program from where the budget is being seeded should not be omitted.

The detailed exercise for a cover letter may seem time-consuming, but it is an essential requirement for all grant applications. Especially if it can draw the attention of the grant agency, then the task is complete [3].

10.2.6 Concluding Formatting the Cover Letter

Always end the cover letters positively, such as "I eagerly await your response". If one's company institute has a managing director who is held responsible for all operations, then the manager signs the letter along with the applicant. The idea is to make the letter sound upbeat and thankful, but this is not required.

10.2.6.1 Tips and Mistakes to Avoid Once Writing a Cover Letter

To complete the proposal, one can personalise and professionalise the cover letter. Revision before clicking submit online or sending hard copies is essential. As mentioned above, if the applicant has a co-worker re-read the letter and proposal, it will help to improve the content from their opinion. It is challenging to get good feedback sometimes, so one has to revise the same again, but once someone obtains good suggestions and revises, check typographical errors, as they are legendary typos that become permanent, for example, misplaced punctuation marks. It is fruitful to have the team's opinion. Hence it is always better to feel free to seek help from the larger community. Send a sample suggestion page to as many people as possible and collect feedback.

Complete the grant form to ensure the cover letter's dates and main grant request match. In the header, the cover letter must utilise a single space and allow a gap between the addresses. Care should be taken that one should not file the grant application with a particular date different from one on the cover letter. For example, a grant application has a date of Aug 29, and the cover letter is on Dec 27. All other related files as well should have synchronous dates.

10.2.6.2 The Format of the Letter

Make letters single-spaced with standard fronts of 11 to 12 in document software. Dual space means one has less room to write the information required. However, the thing does not imply that the spaces between paragraphs should be removed. Allow the letter format enough space to make it presentable. It is essential to leave roughly three gaps for signatures before the end of the letter and then space to type your name.

Send Cover Letter in "Printable Document Format" PDF. If applicants are emailing the grant proposal or uploading the same to the website, preferably always send PDF unless otherwise stated in the grant form. The foundation or organisation may offer to sign the document digitally. Also, PDF files are protected from malware, unlike other text files. The PDF will not only look competent but will impress in the eyes of those funding more technologically advanced grants.

10.2.7 The Significant Aspect of Cover Letter can be Summarised in a Few Significant Facts

1. Cover Letter serves for—Introduction of the "Principal Investigators" and "Organisation" he belongs to the appropriate persons at "Grant Agencies".
2. Cover letter gives a brief of the project, highlighting the main title of the project that needs to be mentioned to the grant agency.
3. A small line about the objective project and outcomes proposed project and its significance is another crucial aspect that has to be incorporated into the letter.
4. The other important aspect is why the particular grant agency was chosen. The letter should indicate which program of the grant agencies the investigators were applying to and how the research project is an ideal match for the grant agency's mandate, mission, and program goals.
5. The cover letter should also mention any previous correspondence with the grant agency, if any between them, primarily if it was related to the same topic or project.
6. A point that must never be omitted is if the grant agency in question has previously granted the principal investigators or their host organisation any financial assistance or grant award to where the cover letter is being sent.
7. The cover letter is the most indispensable tool to establish the credibility and authenticity of the "Principal Investigators" and "Organisation" (Fig. 10.1). The cover letter should always be brief, articulate, and focused, with a signature seal

Fig. 10.1 Cover letter and abstract are primary documents that are reviewed first; hence due importance should be given

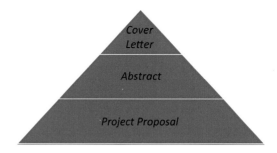

as the complete address for further correspondence if available. The grammar and spellchecked are not optional but essential.

10.3   Abstract for Grant Proposal

The abstract is an essential part of any proposal. The initial impression about the project is built based on how the "Abstract" defines the scope of work, its objectives, outcomes, and novelty. As a separate entity in itself, the abstract defines the proposal. Thus, the abstract primary role is to signify the importance of the work to the grant agency.

10.3.1 Significance of Abstract

The significance of one work, the hypothesis and critical aspects of project objectives, the processes to be followed to achieve the objectives, and the possible effect of the work should all be summarised in the abstract. Though it appears first, the abstract should be finalised most articulately because it serves as a succinct description of the project.

Often the project abstract is the first thing, and the only thing that some senior reviewers like a board of directors grant agency or the senior managers read. In the decision-making meetings, abstracts create the first immersion, which sometimes becomes the final impression for the grant agency officials. Hence due diligence needs to be provided for abstract writing.

The sponsor's specifications determine the length. The abstract grant length usually ranges from up to half to two pages. Most abstracts are limited to 30–50 lines as the maximum as per grant agency format.

10.3.2 Salient Features of How to Write an Abstract

Re-read the project proposal before initiating the abstract writing. As one's goes forward, make a quick overview of the essential features of one's project.

Table 10.3 What exactly is an abstract?

• An abstract is a shortened version of a lengthier piece of writing that emphasises the main points discussed
• Clearly summarises the subject and breadth of the writing and provides an abridged overview of the writing's contents

The main point is how we could convey each of the following abstract components (given by the grant agencies National Institute Health USA or other funding organisations worldwide) in less than one word.

The abstract should explain the unique features of the proposal; specific goals, objectives, or hypotheses; the importance of the proposed study; in line with the funding agency's mission; unique features; methodology (steps) used; expected results;

assessment methods; project background.

- What impact the findings will have on other fields of research.
- The essential feature of the annotations is that they should be brief and provide the main reasoning and project outcomes (Tables 10.3 and 10.4).

If the grant application requires information additional than that listed above, keep these elements in mind. Make notes to examine the proposal without looking at the project report. The exercise will sometimes help find what is missing in the proposal; postulating on an abstract opens new avenues for research project proposals. Sometimes it is imperative to take the help of online software tools. Many online courses and software are good examples of an online writing tool (OWT) [4].

10.3.3 Consider the Essential Project Elements and Norms of Application

One essential thing is not to replicate in the abstract any of the proposed methods work done so far. Otherwise, sometimes we have too much data to handle. However, follow the standards set by the grant agency, including essential elements of information from the project also formatting issues such as the font size format in the grant proposal application [4, 5].

Review the draft according to OWT, correct deficiencies in organisation or clarity, remove unnecessary information, add missing vital points, remove unnecessary words, and ensure that paragraphs are grammatically correct [5, 6]. Each sentence must be annotated and have to be self-explanatory. Abstracts play a significant role in deciding whether to apply or not, as they form the reader's first impression of the work. The abstract speaks in favour of the topic, giving the reader the first impression of the request and serving as a summary, often making a final

Table 10.4 The significance of abstract

1	What are the benefits of an abstract?	• Aids the readers in deciding whether or not to read a complete article • Aids the readers in deciding whether or not to read the entire article • Assist readers and researchers in recalling significant results on a topic • Assist readers in comprehending the text by highlighting key points before reading the entire document
2	What are the essential factors one needs to consider?	• Background: A simple sentence or two to set the tone for the piece • Aims: One or two phrases stating the work's goal • Method(s): A phrase or two describing what was (or will be) done • Outline the significant findings (or what you intend to achieve with the research) in one or two words • Conclusions: One sentence summarises the research's most important outcome—what do the findings imply? What will be done with them?
3	What should an abstract inform us:	• Why was the study or project carried out? (Or what are the inspirations or needs for undertaking the project/study?) • What did you do, and how? (What will you do? How?) • What did you find? (What do you expect to find?) • What do the findings mean?
4	When drafting an abstract, keep these suggestions in mind:	• Go over your article or proposal again to abstract it • Look for the article or proposal's goal, methodology, scope, findings, conclusions, and suggestions • Keep the titles and table of contents in mind when composing your abstract • Write a rough draught without looking back at the work once you have completed reviewing it—what do the results mean? What are your plans for them?

5	What it is that you are abstracting	• Do not just copy essential sentences as it ends up with too much or too little data
		• Freshly rephrase information rather than relying on the way it was expressed
		• Revise the rough draft for:
		  – Fix organisational flaws
		  – Improve point-to-point transitions
		  – Remove extraneous material
		  – Make sure it is thorough and correct
		  – Eliminate wordiness
		  – Fix grammar, spelling, and punctuation mistakes
		  – Make sure it has written in the same tone as the paper

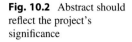
Fig. 10.2 Abstract should reflect the project's significance

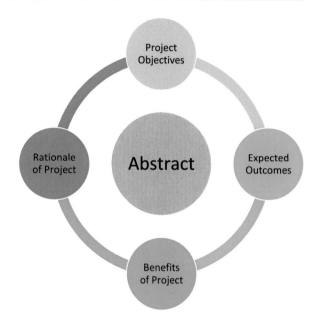

impression on the reader. Some reviewers, such as members of the grant agency board of directors who vote on the final funding decision, only read the abstract.

As a result, it is the proposal's single most crucial component. The length of the abstract is determined by the suggestions of grant agencies and should be strictly followed [7].

The abstract should outline the significance (necessity) of the work, the hypotheses and critical objectives of the project, the processes to be followed to attain the goal, and the work's possible effect on conveying the proposal's essential meaning. The abstract should be written first, but, like the proposal summary, it should be modified last (Fig. 10.2).

10.4   Conclusion

The importance of the cover letter and abstract stems from the fact that they are the first impression of the grant agency; hence, they have to be allocated equal importance in addition to the grant application itself. A well-written "Cover letter" and "Abstract" are the first steps to opening the doors of a grant agency for the application.

Revision and correction are essential. Abstract and cover letter are the cornerstone of a good application, so the time allocated to the composition and multiple revisions are required. Using the few promising modalities and tips we mentioned, every investigator and organisation can compose an appropriate "Cover Letter and Abstract" that correctly highlights the merit of the grant application. Thus a well-written "Cover Letter and Abstract" help the grant agencies take notice of novel research concepts that get reviewed and accepted for the grant award.

Case Scenario and Case Study

A Research Foundation based in a Teaching Hospital supported the clinical faculty to develop their innovations into new novel therapies for indications that do not have good treatment regimens. After obtaining essential data on their innovation from pilot research projects, the research group's Principal Investigators are encouraged to apply for extramural grants. The sample cover letter and abstract here are from such a research project.

Sample Letter
Date: Month/Date/Year
To
Mr S
Director
National Council of Medical Research
New Delhi
India
Dear Sir

Subject: Application for Grant for funds for Novel Treatment for Reducing Mortality in Acute Sepsis, acute post-operative open infected wounds and non-healing ulcers of diabetic foot.

We are applying to your esteemed organisation's program for clinical trials. We have developed a novel treatment that increases the chances of survivability of patients suffering from acute sepsis and post-operative wounds as well non healing ulcers of diabetic foot.

Foremost, I will like to introduce to you that our Institute and Research Foundation is a federally recognised government institution with the mandate to carry out clinical trials and innovative research on human health. I am a senior faculty and clinician specialising in infectious diseases with over 30 years of clinical research and patient care at our tertiary Hospital and Research Institute.

Enclosed with this application are brief details about our organisation and my research experience. Our organisation conducts three years around 150 clinical trials from Phase I/II to Phase 4 are completed around our 35 super speciality hospitals across the country. The hospital I work in has a medical college and a research institute.

I have more than 50 Publications in my field of work, and my recent publication this year. I have secured research grants to carry out the pilot studies on the given topic that I am applying for to your grant agency for an additional grant larger clinical trial.

The preclinical and limited clinical trial results have been published, and I have shared the same with you in the application. We are also manufacturing the new formulation in GMP grade on a large scale with our collaborators in the pharmaceutical sector.

Since our formulation in question is made from a combination of natural nutraceuticals based on substances being used routinely in patients, we have been allowed by the national regulatory authority and our ethical board to carry out our proposed trial. Also, all preclinical and clinical trials have yielded no adverse effects.

The standard operating procedures to date are not as effective in preventing deaths from sepsis as well amputation in diabetic foot in significant number patients. The method proposed here is a unique, novel concept that brings hope to patients with high mortality rates. I am providing all the details in the protocol along with the grant application for your review and feedback.

Based on our initial results in an observational pilot study, we believe that a more extensive trial can now be conducted to take this project forward.

With your organisation's grant support, I believe that our institute can take this project to a logical conclusion. Your organisation's record for support for such novel research under your 'Innovators scheme award' in the last quarter century has been a boon for cutting-edge research. It has brought about new health products to the public.

Our concept matches your organisation's "Innovators scheme grant" application mandate. We have enclosed the required budget, plan, and rationale for conducting the clinical trial.

Hence we are looking forward to your positive response.

With best regards

Professor Dr C

Signature with seal

Prof and Senior Surgeon and Infectious Disease consultant

SA Research Foundation

New Delhi

India

The treatment of non-healing ulcers of the foot in diabetes patients remains a significant challenge. Repeated debridement and recurrent infections lead to amputation of the lower limb, disability, and loss of life. To treat infected diabetic foot ulcers, using antibiotics and other standard methods in clinical practice to control the infection in these patients is complex. It is often met with repeated failures in cases of patients. The study proposes a novel method of using a carrier molecule impregnated with antibiotics that will be delivered at the local site of infection, and dressing will be done using a novel scaffold that is impervious to dust and water resistant.

The patient will be observed, and treatment will be carried out until the infection is eliminated and complete wound healing occurs. The patient would be followed up periodically every 3 months up to 1 year to check for recurrence of infection. The method is simple and easy to apply, and it eliminates the bacteria at the site of infection and heals wounded areas. This single-arm observational study is proposed on 35 patients after Institutional EC clearance and obtaining intramural funding. The methodology will be carried out on diabetic patients for which the selection criteria have been clearly outlined. The outcome measures will be complete healing of wounds, abolition of recurrent infection, and the avoidance of amputations in diabetes patients. The method can be utilised in variety of indication for saving patient post-operative local infection and sepsis. We also propose to carry observational study in 24 postoperative patients suffering from sepsis and post-operative infection. The clinical trial would open new treatment regimen to obtain substantial clinical outcomes in saving lives.

1. State the pros and cons of the letter and abstract by the scientist to the grant agency? How can you improve upon the letter?
2. Is the innovation mentioned in the letter invoke the interest of the reader? Why or why not?
3. If you are a director of a grant agency, what will be your reply to this reader and why?

References

1. Barker R, Rattihalli RR, Field D. How to write a good research grant proposal. Symp Res Paediatr Child Health. 2016;26(3–6):105–9. https://coek.info/pdf-how-to-write-a-good-research-grant-proposal-b285625bbac4c32a4db2be9ef951e00b52167.html
2. Floersch B. What is a grant proposal? Grants as advocacy, not just asking. 2013. https://www.tgci.com/what-grant-proposal. https://www.tgci.com/sites/default/files/pdf/WhatisaGrant-051316-bf.pdf.
3. Cunningham K. Beyond boundaries: developing grant writing skills across higher education institutions, volume LI, number 2, Society of Research Administrators International. USA. https://www.srainternational.org/blogs/srai-jra1/2020/09/29/beyond-boundaries-developing-grant-writing-skills. Accessed 28 Dec 2021.
4. Udemy Grant Writing Courses. https://www.udemy.com/topic/grant-writing/. Accessed 28 Dec 2021.
5. Porter R. Why academics have a hard time writing good grant proposals. J Res Adm. 2007;38(2):37–43. https://files.eric.ed.gov/fulltext/EJ1152279.pdf
6. Essential Online Writing Tools to Help Improve Your Content. https://www.searchenginejournal.com/online-writing-tools/235859/.
7. The University of Iowa Grant writing tools. https://dsp.research.uiowa.edu/grant-writers-tools.

Surveillance Plan and Site Visit: Roles and Rights of the Researcher and the Funding Agency

11

Prasanth Ganesan and Luxitaa Goenka

There's no harm in hoping for the best as long as you're prepared for the worst

Stephen King

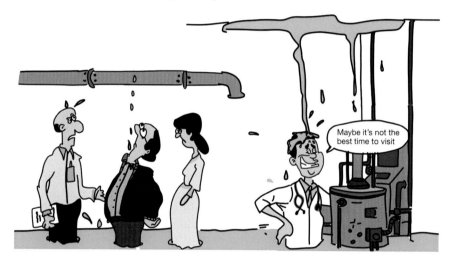

Surveillance plan and site visit

Objectives

This chapter aims to help researchers understand the processes involved in site visits and prepare for them by answering the following questions:

P. Ganesan (✉) · L. Goenka
Department of Medical Oncology, Jawaharlal Institute of Postgraduate Medical Education and Research (JIPMER), Pondicherry, India

© The Author(s), under exclusive license to Springer Nature Singapore Pte Ltd. 2023
S. C. Parija, V. Kate (eds.), *Grant writing for medical and healthcare professionals*, https://doi.org/10.1007/978-981-19-7018-4_11

- Why would the granting agency want to do a site visit?
- How should a researcher prepare for a surveillance and site visit?
- How to make the site visit useful for the researcher as well as the funding agency?

11.1 Introduction

Funding agencies may undertake a site visit to convince themselves about the suitability of a site for funding approval. Additional "surveillance visits" may happen *after* the funds have been approved and the project has commenced. Surveillance visits help the funding agencies to understand the progress of the project. They ensure that the funds are being utilized as per the objectives of the project. The funding agency usually obtains funds for disbursal from multiple donors/government agencies and are themselves answerable as to their proper utilization. These visits help to document that the requirements are being met [1].

The funding agency may directly undertake the visits for evaluation and review. Sometimes, site visits are outsourced to an external agency. These professional agencies have appropriately trained and experienced personnel who perform the assessment on behalf of the funding agency and prepare a report. The visits may be undertaken for evaluation of clinical studies as well as for nonclinical projects [1]. The specific components of monitoring may differ (Tables 11.1 and 11.2).

The recommendations from a site evaluation will often determine whether a grant will be approved for a particular site/researcher. It will also ensure the continuation of the grant if the researcher can satisfy the objectives and demonstrate their achievement. The surveillance visits are an opportunity for the grantee to demonstrate new issues that may have come up during the project. This may help the grantee to justify requirements for additional time, funds, or human resources. The researcher/site would be best served by having a standard operating procedure (SOP) document to be followed for such visits (Table 11.3).

Table 11.1 Monitoring activities for clinical studies and trials

Component	Description
Facilities	Space for personnel to conduct the activities, monitoring, consenting
	Internet connection
	Support from institution
	GCP-trained personnel
	Laboratory facilities such as centrifuge, deep freezer, refrigerators
	Accredited laboratories
	Storage of investigational product
Documents	Ethics committee constitution, Standard operating procedures (SOPs) of the committees and the site activities, registration with regulatory bodies (CDSCO and DHR)
	Trial document storage/archiving facility
Financial	SOPs for financial processes
	Dedicated accounts management process for research funds
Quality management	SOPs for ensuring quality in conduct of trials
	Internal audit SOPs, frequencies, training logs for personnel involved in trial activities

Table 11.2 Monitoring activities for nonclinical research (pure laboratory) projects

Component	Description
Lab manual	Lab manuals with regular updates Shipment of laboratory items: when did the shipment take place, proof of receipt of the items, data on temperature monitoring (and if needed, humidity monitoring) during shipment of items via a temperature logger
Equipment	The general conditions of the laboratory equipment Check that every piece of equipment has an up-to-date SOP Annual calibration of laboratory equipment and record of calibrations Annual maintenance of laboratory equipment and record of maintenance Equipment inventory is in place for the equipment in the lab The logbook is in place to record if equipment is out of order, together with the actions taken and the outcome If equipment is out of order, this is clearly labeled on the machine
Training	The monitor should ensure that all the laboratory personnel are trained in • Good laboratory practice (GLP) • Trained in the use of instruments
Safety practices	Check that all biological specimens are handled as described in the applicable SOPs (e.g., biosafety) Fire alarms are in place Main switches of equipment are switched off when not in use Proper handling of harmful or dangerous chemicals
Disposal of waste	Check that the laboratory is clean, if the benches are disinfected daily, and if the required personal protection is used (lab coats, gloves, masks, etc.) Check that a site-specific procedure for waste management is in place and is correctly applied Check if the procedure for the management of expired products is correctly applied

Table 11.3 Components of a standard operating procedure document to be followed for site visits

Component	Description
Purpose	Describe the purpose of the SOP
Procedure	Describe the timing, the objectives of such visits Describe the personnel who have to be available for a visit
Preparing for a site visit	Describe each of the components which will be evaluated during a site visit in terms of how they should be prepared. Assign responsibility for each component (preparation and review) – Manpower – Equipment – Documents
Schedule of site visits	How to create a schedule and ensure the visit is carried on as per the schedule
Prepare a pre-site visit checklist	Describe the important components. This may be specific for each project

11.2 What Would Be Evaluated in a Site Visit?

The agency may use the site visit to evaluate a particular site's capabilities objectively. For example, the agency may verify infrastructure and space availability, specific equipment claimed to be present, or check the physical records of previous projects claimed to have been conducted. Subjective impressions gathered from the on-site interviews with the PI, and other site staff may also influence the decision to fund the project [2].

11.2.1 Initial Visit (Before Funding)

The following aspects may be evaluated (the exact activities may be dependent on the quantum and type of funding) [3, 4]
1. The overall capability of the organization
   (a) Space, infrastructure, workforce as a whole.
   (b) Administrative organization of the grantee Institution, including financial workflow.
   (c) Support provided to similar projects in the past from the grantee organization.
   (d) Financial capacity of the grantee institution.
       This may include looking at the overall operating budget, sources of revenue, sustenance of operations, and support for research projects.
   (e) Purchase procedures for equipment, timelines for procurement.
   (f) May include interviews with the head of the Institution to understand their view of the proposed project.
       • May enquire about how the administration perceives the project would benefit the Institution.
       • What would be the challenges from the administration's perception.
       • Sustenance of the project in the future after the funding is discontinued from the agency.
       • The commitment of the Institution to support the project may be directly verified.
2. Human resources
   (a) The agency may verify the employment records of staff claimed to be available in the Institution who may be part of the proposed project.
   (b) Direct interviews with the staff to understand their capabilities (qualification, experience, communication skills, problem-solving capacities, workload).
   (c) Duration of employment.
   (d) Subjective inputs from the staff and their perception of the proposed project and its future in the Institution.
3. Physical infrastructure
   (a) Location
       For example, for a project involving clinical material, the location of the hospital may be essential to attract a particular type of patient.

Table 11.4 List of documents to be maintained by the researcher (master file)

Document	Requirement	
	Initial	Surveillance
Staff related		✔
– Training records		
– Attendance		
– Personal information		
– Recruitment-related files		
Regulatory	✔	✔
– Scientific committee		
– Ethics approval		
– Other agency approval documents		
Financial records		✔
– Grant letter		
– Bank statements		
– Bills and invoices		
– UC SOE audited copies		
Equipment related		✔
– Purchase record		
– Maintenance information		
Communication with funding agency	✔	✔
For human participation		✔
Recruitment details (maybe a separate file)		
– Consent documents (if human participation is present)		
– Adverse event reports (for drug trials)		
– Source documents access		
For laboratory studies		✔
– Consumable purchase and utilization records		
– Laboratory manuals		
– Experiment notes		
– Calibration certificates for equipment		
SOPs may be required for the project and for the site	✔	✔

(b) Space

The physical space claimed to be part of the project may be assessed for existing buildings. For projects where new building construction is supported, the area for the same must be demonstrated.

(c) Equipment

Physical verification of equipment that is claimed to be present. The facilities available for equipment to be placed (e.g., UPS connection/24-h-air-conditioning may be required for some types of equipment) has to be demonstrated.

4. Previous records/experience with the conduct of projects (Table 11.4)

This may include checking the grant letters, project completion reports, utilization certificates, ethics committee approval certificates, etc. This may convince the agency about the capability of the Institution to conduct similar projects.

11.2.2 Surveillance Visit (During the Conduct of the Project)

1. Utilization of the funds
   (a) Physical verification of invoices, bills of purchase, purchase, and payment procedures.
   (b) Payment of staff salaries: verify the attendance registers/electronic records, interview the staff, dates of recruitment/resignation, etc.
2. Achievement of the objective(s)
   The agency may look at the records to check whether the project's proposed objectives have been realized. For example, in a project involving a clinical study, they may look at the patient records and the consent forms to verify the number of participants involved in the study.
3. Equipment(s) bought with the funds and their status
   (a) Physical verification of the equipment and its functional status.
   (b) Purchase records (whether proper procedures have been followed during the purchase—for costly equipment, whether tenders were floated and the lowest quoting vendor was chosen).
   (c) Maintenance/calibration records of the equipment.
4. Human resources
   (a) Recruitment procedures: whether the recruitment procedures recommended by the funding agency (if any) were followed. The records of advertisement for the posts, interview minutes, the announcement of results, mark sheets, and other documents may be verified.
   (b) Training of the recruited workforce.
      • Usual institution training: Employee safety, fire response, and other training(s) imparted to all employees of the Institution.
      • Training specific to the project: Records of these training(s) should be maintained.
      • Training manuals/SOPs.
      • Other training materials imparted to the staff.
   (c) Periodic assessment reports of the staff and the renewal of contractual employment-related documents.
   (d) Leave records.
   (e) Records of any disciplinary action or termination of any employee in a project.
5. Documentation (Table 11.4)
   All project-related files must be maintained. In addition to specific documentation about fund use, workforce recruitment, and purchase procedures as indicated above, this may also include the following:
   (a) Application and grant letters.
   (b) Email communication with the funding agency.
   (c) MOUs/Agreements which are part of the project.
6. Problems faced and solutions
   (a) *Problems faced by the PI/Institution:* In addition to verifying the conduct of the project, the agency may also enquire about the challenges faced by the PI. This is an opportunity for the PI to highlight issues and demonstrate them

directly to the funding agency. This may help to justify delays in the project and ask for additional support from the agency.

(b) *Solution(s):* Often, professional agencies conduct the surveillance visits, and they may suggest solutions for some of the issues faced by the PI in the conduct of the project.

11.3 Role of the Researcher. How to Prepare for a Site/Surveillance Visit?

The researcher will have to understand the various activities which are mentioned in the previous section, which may be part of the site visits. It would be best for the researcher to communicate with the funding agency to understand their plan for the visit and have an agenda prepared (Table 11.5) [3, 4].

Table 11.5 Checklist for preparing for a site/surveillance visit [4]

Item	Yes/no
1. Email communication with funding agency confirming date and time of visit	
2. Clear agenda for visit agreed with the agency (a) Time of visit and visit plan (b) What physical inspections do they need to complete? (c) Whom all does the agency need to interview? (d) Is an interview with the head of the institution planned?—take an appointment and confirm (e) What specific records do they need to see (keep them prepared)?	
3. Records are available for review and are updated, signed, and checked	
4. Staff need to be available, and only emergency leaves are allowed	
5. Prepare the staff for a visit and ensure they are capable of responding appropriately during the evaluation visits (a) What questions may be asked and how to respond? (b) Training records	
6. Equipment purchase and maintenance records (a) Equipment(s) bought through project funds available for check (b) Records of purchase process and payment (c) Other equipment used for the project available in the Institution (d) Maintenance and calibration records (e) Accreditation records (where applicable)	
8. Have a list of issues to be discussed with the agency/problems which need to be sorted	
9. Are you asking for additional time, funds, and workforce? If yes, keep the justification for these ready for discussion/inspection	
10. Documents about the actual conduct of the project (inform consent forms, laboratory notes) (a) Records for previous projects to demonstrate the capability (b) All documents signed and dated (c) Original documents whenever possible	
11. Ensure that light refreshments are available for the inspector but nothing extravagant is to be provided or arranged for. This can be discussed with the inspector and if they prefer to make their own arrangements then respect their wishes	

11.3.1 Before the Visit

The following needs to be done before planning the visit with the agency
1. **Websites:** If the agency is not aware about your organization's capability, the first step would be to check the website (before planning a site visit). So it is essential to make sure that the website is up to date and well-maintained and highlights critical achievements and capabilities of your department as well as the Institution.
2. **Agenda:** They may communicate and want specific information through emails. Respond honestly to these requests and provide accurate and verifiable information. Communicate with the agency to understand what exactly they would be looking for from the researcher and the organization. If the visit involves an interview with the institution's head or some other administrative staff, fix the appointment time well in advance to ensure their availability.

11.3.2 During the Visit

11.3.2.1 Documents
Make sure all physical copies are available. Can communicate with the sponsor before the visit to understand their needs and keep these ready.

11.3.2.2 Presentation
Make a good case for funding—highlight the unique aspects of the site. A good presentation must highlight the following elements:

(a) What makes the site special?
(b) Specific infrastructure is available which will help in the conduct of the project.
(c) Specific capabilities of the staff relevant to the project.
(d) Previous track record (show evidence).
(e) Challenges can be presented honestly, along with plans to tackle them when they arise.

11.3.2.3 Site Tour
The visit often involves a tour of the facility. This must be planned and organized beforehand. Ensure that the visit doesn't happen on a holiday, or on a day when the PI has no free time. It is important for the PI to directly interact with the team coming for the evaluation visit.

(a) Involve the other staff.
(b) Keep the premises well organized and neat.
(c) If the PI cannot spend the entire time with the funding evaluation team, ensure that suitably trained staff are available to conduct at least part of the tour.

11.3.2.4 Surveillance Visit

In this situation, the funding has been approved and the project has commenced. The agency wants to understand whether the funds are being appropriately used and the objectives achieved. The items mentioned in Sect. 11.3.2 must be prepared and ready (also see Table 11.5).

11.4   Rights of the Researcher

Even though site visits are an essential component of the decision-making process for agencies involved in funding, there are certain rights that the researcher can maintain.

1. **Advance information**
   The researcher should be informed sufficiently in advance about the visit to prepare the site for a visit. It would be desirable to have a mutually agreed schedule/agenda for a visit.
2. **Opportunity to explain shortcomings/deficiencies in the site/conduct of the project**
   There may be explanations for the non-achievement of specific goals/milestones by the researcher. The agency must hear these. Also, the researcher may have contingency plans in place.
3. **Time to prepare the reports**
   They must be given sufficient time to provide a report about the conduct of the project.
4. **Confidentiality of records**
   Certain patient-related documents, study findings, as well as staff records may be considered confidential. The researcher may decide not to share some of these with the finding agency.

11.5   Role of the Funding Agency

The funding agency spends effort and money in conducting a visit. It is important to plan this carefully to make it meaningful. Key components of making a site visit useful to the funding agency are [3, 4]:

1. Prepare well—communicate the goals in advance. Send an email/letter communication to the PI to document the above plans and a clear agenda.
2. Ensure that sufficient time is given to the site for preparation and a clear agenda is circulated and key personnel are available.
3. Decide on the site visit team—number of members needed, the expertise required to evaluate specific components of the project.

4. Make sure that the grantee understands that the visit is to enhance and improve the project as a whole and need not be perceived as a stressful experience.
5. Encourage the grantee to discuss the challenges faced and if possible, provide solutions.
6. The timing of the site visit should be such that it does not impede the workflow of an organization.
7. If the inspector is from outside (outsourced) organization, clear communication with the granting agency to understand their requirement for the inspection.
8. Meet with the PI and project staff and tour the facility to understand the objectives.
9. Within a prespecified time (usually 1–2 weeks), a site visit report is prepared and shared with the grantee and the funding agency.
   (a) Point by point appraisal as per the original agenda.
   (b) Any additional issues noted during the visit.
   (c) The report should have clear documentation of the positive aspects and achievements of the project as well as shortcomings with the suggestion (s) to modify/overcome issues.
   (d) It would be useful for the report to have action points, prespecified timelines for their achievement, and the designation of responsibility for these activities. This part may be prepared after consultation with the project PI and the funding agency.

11.6 Other Forms of Monitoring

Due to pandemic-induced (or other) restrictions, there may be restrictions in conducting physical visits. Hence, the agency may choose to have other methods of monitoring.

11.6.1 Remote Monitoring

Remote monitoring allows funding agencies to remotely conduct monitoring activities that were previously conducted on-site due to restrictions of the pandemic. Remote monitoring can be done by sharing documents and reports through fax, email, cloud-based file share systems, web-conferencing, or by granting monitors direct access to their electronic medical records (EMR) without sharing confidential information.

11.6.2 Centralized Monitoring

Centralized monitoring involves analytical evaluation carried out by sponsor personnel or representatives at a central location other than the site at which the clinical investigation is being conducted.

11.6.3 Reverse Site Visit

It is not always mandatory that the funding agency should physically visit the site for inspection. In these cases, the grantee may be asked to visit the granting agency to make a presentation to describe their position and clarify issues. This may be termed a "reverse visit." The agenda points may be similar, and the grantee may make his position clear with the help of photographs, videos, and other "soft" documents.

11.7   Conclusion

Site visits and evaluations are integral to large extramurally funded projects. With sufficient awareness and preparedness, these can be handled comfortably. Instead of being a stressful experience, the investigator should look upon these as opportunities to showcase his/her/site's capabilities, and achievements. These are also occasions to audit the processes and apply course corrections where required. The expertise of the funding agency/inspectors can provide valuable inputs for solving problems that arise during the conduct of a study.

Case Scenarios
1. A principal investigator has applied for a project for the development of a registry of adverse events of cancer drugs. This will involve data inputs from 30 different centers across the country. His center will contribute data as well as serve as coordinating center. Funding will involve many crores and will support the software and hardware to host the database, manpower for data entry, and monitoring of the project. The funding agency wants to visit his center to ascertain their capability in coordinating and conducting this project.
   A. How should the PI prepare for this visit?
   B. What are the aspects which the funding agency should be checking so that the project is successful and the money is well spent?
2. Two years into a project, the funding agency wants to do random site visits to assess status of progress. They send an email communication to the PI 1 day before that they are coming for a visit and ask him to be ready with all documents, equipment details, site personnel, and laboratory work records. The PI is busy with department exams on that day and is not in a position to arrange these. How can he respond to this situation? Discuss the pros and cons of the various options given below.

A. The PI has a right to be informed with sufficient notice to prepare and he can inform the funding agency about his inability to cooperate.
B. The PI can inform that some of the records may be available but everything may not be available at short notice and can designate a co-PI or project manager to be with the inspection.
C. The is bound to cooperate with the FA and must postpone the department exam and ensure that the inspection is attended to.

References

1. Site Visits, Grantee SOP. https://www.niaid.nih.gov/research/site-visits-grantee-sop. Accessed 4 Oct 2021.
2. How-To Note: Planning and Conducting Site Visits. Version 3. 2021. https://www.niaid.nih.gov/research/site-visits-grantee-sop. Accessed 4 Oct 2021.
3. The truth about site visits. The Truth About Site Visits | Minnesota Council on Foundations (mcf.org). https://mcf.org/truth-about-site-visits. Accessed 4 Oct 2021.
4. Site visit reports. University of Melbourne. https://students.unimelb.edu.au/academic-skills/explore-our-resources/report-writing/site-visit-reports. Accessed 4 Oct 2021.

Sources of Funding and Acknowledgement: Good Clinical Practice Guidelines

Karthick Subramanian, Avin Muthuramalingam, and Vigneshvar Chandrasekaran

> *No one who achieves success does so without acknowledging the help of others. The wise and confident acknowledge this help with gratitude*
>
> *Alfred North Whitehead*

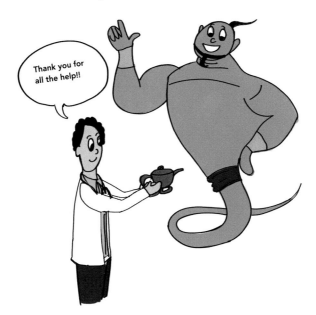

Sources of funding and acknowledgement—good clinical practice guidelines

K. Subramanian (✉) · V. Chandrasekaran
Department of Psychiatry, Mahatma Gandhi Medical College and Research Institute, Sri Balaji Vidyapeeth, Pondicherry, India

A. Muthuramalingam
Department of Psychiatry, Jawaharlal Institute of Postgraduate Medical Education and Research (JIPMER), Karaikal, India

© The Author(s), under exclusive license to Springer Nature Singapore Pte Ltd. 2023
S. C. Parija, V. Kate (eds.), *Grant writing for medical and healthcare professionals*, https://doi.org/10.1007/978-981-19-7018-4_12

Objectives
The chapter aims to address
- The necessity of reporting sources of funding.
- Good Clinical Practice Guidelines on reporting sources of funding.
- Structure and content in reporting funding sources with examples.
- The eligibility for mention under acknowledgements.
- Structure and content of acknowledgements with examples.

12.1 Reporting Sources of Funding

12.1.1 Overview

Successfully winning a grant creates a very much rewarding experience for anyone who painstakingly proceeds with each stage of grant preparation, submission, and follow-up. The positive experience is secondary to the acceptance and appreciation of such efforts [1]. Hence, for all that has become so valuable, one can take time and bask in the success of grant acceptance. It should also be noted that the grant serves benefits not only for the applicant but also for the institution or the agency which has provided the grant. Getting grants, either the first time or in succession brings not just joy but also added responsibility. Because the generosity of the organization or agency must be acknowledged and repaid with quality research, keeping in line with ethical and regulatory norms of the region.

Thanksgiving does not end there. After completion of research, the source of funding and the various members who contributed to the body and conduct of research must be acknowledged in the write-up of the research work.

12.1.2 Expressing Gratitude

To get started, it is accepted to write a personal "thank-you note" to the head of the agency or the person who furnished the grant announcement. The same note can be officially drafted if the funding agency is governmental or government aided.

Several sources, including sponsors, labs, research councils, charities, governing bodies, or industry, can be involved. Assistance from such sources includes financial or similar support. Such sources need to be mentioned in a separate section at the end of the research work.

12.1.3 Reporting Sources of Funding: Why It Is Important?

Reporting the sources of funds usually precedes the acknowledgement section. Also, it helps the funding bodies to track the research output and conclude on the judicious use of the fund. It allows the research institute to know the publication status of the research done using the fund. Finally, it would help fellow researchers know which funding agency to approach for research funds if they are in the same field of scientific research as the investigator [2].

12.1.4   Good Clinical Practice Guidelines: What Does It Say About Sources of Funding?

The sponsor or the funding agency becomes one of the important participants in the Good Clinical Practice (GCP) Guidelines for research [3]. The GCP for research provides a framework for the ethical and moral conduct of research in human studies. In the section, "finance and insurance", GCP states that: [4, 5].

"The information should be available about the sources of economic support (e.g., foundations, private or public funds, sponsor/manufacturer). Likewise, it should be stated how the expenditures should be distributed, e.g., payment to subjects, refunding expenses of the subjects, payments for special tests, technical assistance, purchase of apparatus, a possible fee to or reimbursement of the members of the research team, payment of the investigator/institution, etc.)". It also states that if this is not satisfactorily stated, the following needs to be disclosed: "The financial arrangement between the sponsor, the individual researcher(s)/manufacturer involved, institution and the investigator(s) in case such information is not stated explicitly". Hence, it is clear that the reporting of sources of funding leads to enhanced transparency in the conduct and publishing of research involving human participants.

12.1.5   Funder Registry

The Funder Registry, commonly recognized as FundRef, is a funding source database initiated and maintained by CrossRef®. It helps in differentiating the providers of funded research projects and the persons or bodies in receipt of funding. Donated by Elsevier, the registry is updated every month with records of research funding. Periodic review of the database also ensures that the sources mentioned stand relevant and accurate. Overall, the Funder Registry allows for the easy tracking of funding, especially because funding sources are not always reported in academic publications, and funding bodies are forced to mine data to find which publications have come about as a result of their grants.

12.1.6   Reporting Sources of Funding: Structure and Content

The reporting phrase should encompass the full name of the funding agency and the grant number in square brackets. If more than one funding agency is involved in the study, they should be named consecutively with a semicolon separating them. If more than one grant number exists for the same funding agency, a comma and a space should separate each [6].

Here are some examples:

Example 1 (Author's statement version and single source):
"The author would like to thank the Indian Council of Medical Research [ICMR/XX/2021] for funding the study".

Example 2 (Neutral statement version and more than one source)
"The work was funded by the Indian Council of Medical Research [ICMR/XX/2021]; and the Department of Science and Technology [DST/YY/2021]".

Example 3 (First-person version)
"I would like to submit my thanks to the Department of Health Research [DHR/XX/2020, DHR/YY/2021] for funding the research".

12.1.7 Reporting Sources of Funding: Special Mention

There can be various instances where the primary investigator wishes to acknowledge the role(s) of a specific person(s) in acquiring the grant. The researcher can then make subjective statements of appreciation to a particular member or group of the funding agency who helped in approval [7].

Example
"I would like to thank the *Director* of the Indian Council of Medical Research for approving the grants for the conduct of the study".

There can also be situations where two or more funding agencies have participated in the research endeavour leading to multiple independent contributions to the research. Hence, it is advised that the researcher mentions the specific contribution the funding agency has made:

Example (First-person version, single source, more than one grant)
"I would like to submit my thanks to the Department of Health Research [DHR/XX/2020, DHR/YY/2021] *for funding the ELISA reagents used* in the research".

12.1.8 Reporting Sources of Funding: Some Cautions

While being generous enough to list the sources of funding and acknowledging their roles in research, as part of the good ethical practices in research, it is important to keep certain things in consideration before one documents the acknowledgement. It is essential to put disclaimers explicitly to avoid undue research-related implications to the funding agency or the organization.

Common disclaimers
"The funding agencies above mentioned has no role in the design, collection of data and interpretation of the study results"
"*The funding agency was not involved* in the establishment of this article, and this article should not be attributed to the agency or any person connected with the agency"
"The *views expressed are those of the author*(s) and not necessarily those of the agency"

Some funding agencies might recommend their research investigators follow certain prescribed formats in writing down the sources of funding section. It will be the responsibility of the researcher to be cognizant of those guidelines and draft the section accordingly.

Finally, errors in the spelling of the funding agencies, entering wrong grant numbers, and forgetting the necessary details of the funding agencies must certainly be avoided. Additionally, a double-check by all the contributing authors can be considered during the proofreading of these aspects [8].

12.2 Writing Acknowledgements

12.2.1 Overview

Research is community-driven and possible with a team of intellectual researchers, proactive administrators, and funders who envisage creating a productive society through scientific research. As a principal investigator of a research study, one is often supported by a team of researchers who serve as co-principal investigators and a good number of peers, staff, logistic managers, lab technicians, institute administrators, and funders. The former is given authorship for the intellectual contribution; the latter is acknowledged for their involvement in propelling the research study. Acknowledgement falls in the line of the reward spectrum, the others being authorship and citation [9]. The author should write the acknowledgement after the discussion section of the scientific study and before the reference, following the instruction of the journal's publishers [10].

12.2.2 Acknowledgements: Whom to Choose?

Acknowledgement in scientific publications expresses the author's gratitude to diverse entities who inspired, funded, supported, and contributed to the study [11]. The author, in this section, can proceed in acknowledging the support from academic perspectives to a personal appreciation of all other forms of non-academic support. The former refers to personnel and entities who supported the research, and the latter refers to people who gave emotional and moral support during the research period. The various contributions which can be considered for acknowledgements are listed in Box 12.1 [7, 10]. It is also important to obtain permission from those persons who are to be acknowledged in work, and preferably they should be in written form [12].

Box 12.1: Criteria for acknowledgements
- Assistance in data collection
- Assistance with writing (not scientific contribution)
- Assistance with proofreading
- Routine technical assistance
- Clerical support (preparation of supporting documents, correspondence, etc.)
- Leadership or guidance support (heads of departments, chairperson of committees, etc.)
- Moral and personal support

12.2.3 Acknowledgements: Structure and Content

Generally, the message about acknowledgements contains the following elements:

Investigator(s) in the first-person or third-person voice—Thanking verb with or without an adjective—Identity of the individual—Type of assistance received

---

Additionally, a few more considerations are important while writing acknowledgements such as
- Full names of all individuals who are being thanked.
- Appropriate salutations.
- Full names of the group/firm/organization.
- A brief statement regarding what kind of help the researcher has received from each individual or the group of individuals, organizations, etc.

12.2.4 Acknowledgements: Examples

- I am deeply grateful to Mr./Ms..xxx... for providing *technical* support.
- We gratefully acknowledge the support of...yyy...in *proofreading* the manuscript.
- The investigators sincerely thank the xxx organization for providing *clerical* support in the conduct of this research work.
- I sincerely submit my gratitude to Prof. yyy for his/her valuable *guidance and moral support* throughout the conduct of this study.

12.3 Conclusion

The formal achievement of a grant is indeed a significant milestone in the process of sponsored research. The funding agency, whether governmental or private, needs to be duly acknowledged by the investigator(s). There are various forms of mentioning the contents related to "source(s) of funding", each having specific relevance. Similarly, the works and contributions of various other people or groups of individuals need to be separately mentioned as "acknowledgement notes" towards the end of the research report. There can be a variety of support involved in the research work ranging from academic to personal support, all of which needs to be mentioned under the "acknowledgement" section. One needs to be judicious, sincere, and yet cautious while writing all the necessary components of "sources of funding" and "acknowledgements". A good acknowledgement seals the successful process of a grant transforming into fruitful research work.

Case Scenarios

1. Ms. K, a PhD scholar who has finished her thesis has to acknowledge the funding agency in her thesis manuscript and in her proposed publications. What items she need to consider before proceeding for acknowledging the funding body?
   - Identify the source of funding (including the correct title of the funding body) from the Funder Registry or from documents of correspondence received from the agency.
   - Prepare on the structure and content of funding acknowledgement statement depending on the number of agencies involved.
   - Identify the key persons or personnel involved in the funding process and special mention can be prepared.
   - Has to mention the involvement or non-involvement of the funding agency in the design, process, and conduct of the project.
2. When a research scholar thinks that there are many significant persons who aided in the research apart from those directly involved (guides, funding agencies, co-investigators), how to include an appropriate "acknowledgements" section?

- Most importantly, the funding agency needs to be mentioned.
- Personnel who contributed to the data synthesis, draft preparation, clerical assistance, leadership or guidance, moral or personal support shall be mentioned.
- Include the full names with appropriate salutations and mention the type of contribution rendered towards the planning or conduct of the research project.

References

1. Karsh E, Fox AS. The only grant-writing book you'll ever need. New York: Hachette UK; 2019. p. 402.
2. Funding Acknowledgements—Clarivate [Internet]. http://wokinfo.com/products_tools/multi disciplinary/webofscience/fundingsearch/. Accessed 27 Sept 2021.
3. Vijayananthan A, Nawawi O. The importance of good clinical practice guidelines and its role in clinical trials. Biomed Imaging Interv J. 2008;4(1):e5.
4. Castelino LJ, Narayanan VA, Fernandes SD, Kumar P, Sandeep DS. Good clinical practices: an Indian perspective. Res J Pharm Technol. 2018;11(7):3209–15.
5. Indian Council of Medical Research. National ethical guidelines for biomedical and health research involving human participants. New Delhi: Indian Council of Medical Research; 2017.
6. How to Cite Funding in Research—Charlesworth Author Services [Internet]. https://www. cwauthors.com/article/how-to-cite-funding-in-research. Accessed 27 Sept 2021.
7. Paul-Hus A, Desrochers N. Acknowledgements are not just thank you notes: a qualitative analysis of acknowledgements content in scientific articles and reviews published in 2015. PLoS One. 2019;14(12):e0226727.
8. Rigby J. Systematic grant and funding body acknowledgement data for publications: new dimensions and new controversies for research policy and evaluation. Res Eval. 2011;20(5): 365–75.
9. Costas R, van Leeuwen TN. Approaching the "reward triangle": general analysis of the presence of funding acknowledgments and "peer interactive communication" in scientific publications. J Am Soc Inf Sci Technol. 2012;63(8):1647–61.
10. Peh WCG, Ng KH. Authorship and acknowledgements. Singap Med J. 2009;50(6):563–5.
11. Tang L, Hu G, Liu W. Funding acknowledgment analysis: queries and caveats. J Assoc Inf Sci Technol. 2017;68(3):790–4.
12. Liesegang TJ, Bartley GB. Footnotes, acknowledgments, and authorship: toward greater responsibility, accountability, and transparency. Ophthalmology. 2014;121(12):2297–8.

Writing a Grant Proposal for a Collaborative Study

13

Savio George Barreto

The best ideas emerge when very different perspectives meet

Frans Johansson

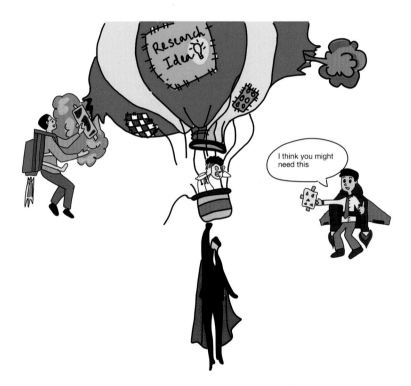

Writing a grant proposal for collaborative study

S. G. Barreto (✉)
Hepatopancreatobiliary and Liver Transplant Unit, Division of Surgery and Perioperative Medicine, Flinders Medical Centre, Adelaide, SA, Australia

College of Medicine and Public Health, Flinders University, Adelaide, SA, Australia

S. C. Parija, V. Kate (eds.), *Grant writing for medical and healthcare professionals*,
https://doi.org/10.1007/978-981-19-7018-4_13

153

Objectives
- Delineate the various roles of collaborators in a collaborative grant proposal.
- Able to set achievable targets with respective timelines when collaborating with multiple individuals.
- Understand the shared responsibility for the outcomes of the project, such as publication and intellectual property.

13.1 Introduction

One of the many concerns in health care has been the uniform lack of ability to translate research into practice within a reasonable time [1]. The traditional "linear" approach of translating research into practice represents an impediment to the process [2]. These early observations, supported by a growing appreciation amongst scientists of the need to engage with other researchers and practitioners with a common goal of enhancing not only the amount and diversity of research but also facilitating its dissemination, have led to a positive revolution of collaboration [3]. Funding agencies, too, have come to realize the importance of collaboration in facilitating the translation of research into practice and are increasingly laying down requirements mandating the elucidation of the plan for dissemination and translation of research as a condition for funding [4].

This requirement from funding agencies has led to researchers now having to actively pursue collaborators and develop collaborations. While collaborating in research brings with it the exciting prospect of "combining powers" (a phrase made famous by the cartoon *Captain Planet and the Planeteers*), it carries with it a unique set of challenges at an individual and institutional level that every researcher needs to be aware of to avoid future discord and disharmony. It is important to approach and interact with collaborators with respect, honesty, and transparency from the outset, and this process begins with planning the grant proposal.

This chapter will provide the reader with an insight into what specific aspects of a collaborative grant proposal need due attention to minimize discord and disharmony and maximize research output and its translation for the betterment of the end-users, namely, the community.

13.2 What Areas in Planning a Collaborative Grant Proposal Warrant Attention?

13.2.1 Communication

Writing a collaborative grant proposal, like any other collaboration, involves the integration of multiple perspectives and the building of consensus [5] when framing the overall aims and objectives. It is, thus, fraught with the potential for disagreements. Clear, honest, and transparent communication is the key to any collaboration since trust forms the basis of any meaningful union between individuals. Maintaining open lines of communication throughout, not only at the time of writing the grant but even during the conduct of the project and dissemination of its findings, is paramount. Researchers and practitioners must endeavor to meet each other in person or virtually (in the context of restrictions imposed by COVID-19) to understand what it is that they are seeking to achieve by this collaboration. Collaboration is a "holistic process" that takes time when building a team—time which may not always be plenty, especially if the period from the date of announcement of grant to the date of closure is short. However, the discussions on the points covered below need to occur before embarking on a collaborative research project.

The team needs to appoint one researcher to lead the cohort as the Chief/Lead Investigator. The chief investigator often (though not always) lands up being the person who initiated the discussion. This person must be mindful of respecting the position and autonomy of the lead investigators from the other teams. The Chief/Lead Investigator maintains the overarching responsibility of preparing and submitting the grant proposal. At the initial meetings, it is important to clarify whether this person and/or their institute will be responsible for reporting to the funding agency and the regulatory bodies and whether they will handle the processes involved in managing potential breaches of the Code of Conduct of research prescribed by the funding agency [6].

13.2.2 Decisions on Principal, Co-, and Other Investigators

It is a healthy practice to clarify the expectations of all the teams involved in the collaboration, as well as their understanding of the individual and institutional roles and responsibilities. This starts with deciding who the Principal and Co-investigators will be, which is generally guided by the extent of contribution to the conceptualization and design of the study, collection of data, its analysis, and interpretation. The roles and responsibilities of every investigator have been covered under the International Conference on Harmonisation Good Clinical Practice guidelines. However, in the event of any difference in opinion amongst investigators, one strategy would be to also refer to the guidelines prescribed by the funding agency. As an example, in Australia, the National Health and Medical Research Council has a Handbook on Research Governance [7] that outlines these roles and responsibilities.

13.2.3 Decisions on the Governance of the Project

The initial discussions between collaborating teams must take into consideration the responsibility surrounding the governance of the project [6]. This would include matters such as who would maintain the overarching responsibilities of informing the ethics committees and funding agencies regarding significant changes to the project, including reporting protocol deviations and serious adverse events, as well as other significant changes to the submitted proposal, including collaborators leaving, or joining, the project, with the attendant issues of stewardship, or control, of the research data generated by that individual and their team. These discussions must also factor in the handling and maintenance of data, as well as the processes of destruction of the data on completion of the study to comply with the requirements of the ethics committee while upholding participant confidentiality. Finally, any conflict of interest on the part of any investigator must be declared to the team and listed clearly in the proposal.

13.2.4 Authorship in Publications Ensuing from the Research

Deciding authorship and its order (especially first and corresponding author) is another area that ought to be discussed at the initial meetings. While it may not always be possible to decide this at the time of writing the proposal, agreeing on the methodology that will be employed represents a healthy strategy, especially when multiple individuals between and even within teams will be doing key, but complementary, aspects of the study. In the absence of a defined strategy by the teams, one objective technique that can be considered is the use of authorship determination and tie-breaker scorecards [8, 9].

13.2.5 Intellectual Property

Intellectual property, protecting the future use of the outcomes of the project, is another significant area that warrants discussion. Having a legally binding, clear agreement in place demonstrating that an Investigator, or the Collaborative group, has rights or permissions to use the outcomes is paramount when one considers the legal implications of not having one. The University of Bristol [10] has published online a simple document to educate researchers on the importance of intellectual property agreements. From a legal perspective, failure to clarify who owns the intellectual property rights and permissions through a contractual agreement could preclude the investigator's ability to do what they wish to with their own data, even if the intellectual property rights are shared. While this is the position in the United Kingdom, it would be worthwhile clarifying the legal remit within the country of the funding agency.

13.2.6 Funding Arrangements

There are a few areas that need to be clarified in relation to funding arrangements. The most important questions to be addressed are:

(a) What funding is already available with one, or more, of the investigators?
(b) What funding is needed to successfully complete the planned study? How will the funds be used (categories)?
(c) Which funding agencies will be approached? Can the funds obtained from the funding agency be used across sites? What are the rules of the funding agency with regard to foreign (another country) collaborators—are they expected to procure their own funding?
(d) How will these funds be divided across sites?
(e) What will be done with the unused funds?

These questions are self-explanatory. Being upfront in terms of seeking answers from them would help create a healthy and supportive environment in the broader group. Additionally, major funding agencies expect these matters to be clarified within the grant proposal.

13.3 Writing the Actual Proposal

Once the collaborative team has tackled all the significant issues listed above, the next important step is to divide the tasks and provide achievable timelines for completing the proposal. The purpose of providing timelines is to permit sufficient time for editing and collation of the main document. Before starting to write the proposal, it is important that the grant writers do the following:

(a) Identify grant opportunities with which your research aligns—this will improve the chances of getting funded.
(b) Read the specific requirements (word and page limits, font size, spacing, etc.) and ensure that these are adhered to.
(c) Pitch the proposal to the aims and mission statement of the funding agency.

The principles of writing a grant are similar to those mentioned in my previous chapter on writing one's thesis [11] (Fig. 13.1). It is the responsibility of the grant writers to ensure that the manuscript is edited to fulfill the requirements listed by the funding agency. Personally, the author would advise grant writers to seek the help of a native speaker to copyedit the document for the language in which the grant is being submitted.

13.4 Conclusion

Collaboration in research presents an exciting opportunity to bring together varied but complementary expertise to help conduct meaningful research with the promise of a higher propensity to translate research into practice. The prospect of collaboration also carries with it the potential for misunderstandings. Addressing key aspects in the collaboration through regular, clear, and transparent communication all

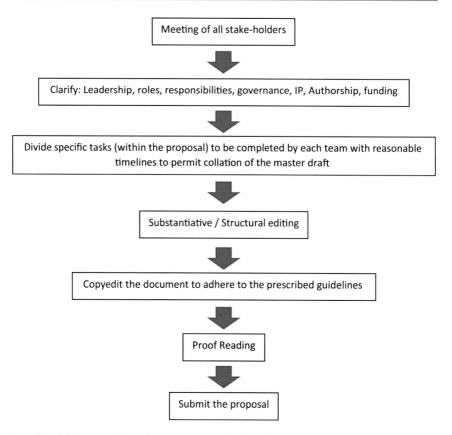

Fig. 13.1 Writing a collaborative grant proposal (*IP* intellectual property)

throughout the project, starting with the discussion that precedes writing the grant, will obviate any risk of disharmony and discord. Attention to detail and pitching the proposal to align with the aims of the funding agency are essential to guarantee success in grant applications.

Case Scenario

John and his team are involved in a multicenter collaborative project with the Chief Investigator based in the United States. The project, which has received significant funding from the National Institute of Health (NIH), involved the use of an experimental drug (compared to a placebo) for treating postoperative paralytic ileus. John had also obtained some seed funding from his own institute, and the project had been approved by the local research ethics committee. One of the test subjects at John's center developed a serious adverse reaction after being administered the drug resulting in the patient being shifted to the intensive care unit. What is John's obligation with regard to reporting the serious adverse event?

1. Just ignore it. No one was sure whether the experimental drug caused the patient's clinical deterioration.
2. Inform the hospital research ethics committee at his own hospital once the patient is discharged from the hospital.
3. Report the reaction as a serious adverse event (SAE) to the local hospital ethics committee as well as to the Chief Investigator, the other Principal Investigators, and the NIH within 24 h of the event.

References

1. McIntyre D. Bridging the gap between research and practice. Camb J Educ. 2005;35(3):357–82.
2. Haines A, Jones R. Implementing findings of research. BMJ. 1994;308(6942):1488–92.
3. Nystrom ME, Karltun J, Keller C, Andersson GB. Collaborative and partnership research for improvement of health and social services: researcher's experiences from 20 projects. Health Res Policy Syst. 2018;16(1):46.
4. Golden-Biddle K, Reay T, Petz S, Witt C, Casebeer A, Pablo A, et al. Toward a communicative perspective of collaborating in research: the case of the researcher-decision-maker partnership. J Health Serv Res Policy. 2003;8(Suppl 2):20–5.
5. Dopke L, Crawley W. Strategies for increasing the efficacy of collaborative grant writing groups in preparing federal proposals. J Res Adm. 2013;44(1):36–61.
6. National Health and Medical Research Council. Collaborative research: a guide supporting the Australian Code for the Responsible Conduct of Research. 2020. https://www.nhmrc.gov.au/sites/default/files/documents/attachments/Collaborative-Research-Guide-20.pdf.
7. Australian Government. National Health and Medical Research Council. Research Governance Handbook: guidance for the national approach to single ethical review. 2011. https://www.nhmrc.gov.au/sites/default/files/documents/reports/research-governance-handbook.pdf.
8. Winston JRB. A suggested procedure for determining order of authorship in research publications. J Couns Dev. 1985;63:515–8.
9. Gaffey A. Determining and negotiating authorship. 2015. http://www.apa.org/science/about/psa/2015/06/determining-authorship.
10. Dunleavy K, Brown E. Intellectual property agreements. A university of Bristol guide for collaboration and knowledge exchange. 2018. http://www.bristol.ac.uk/media-library/sites/brigstow/documents/UoB%20IP%20Guide_Final_web%20ready%20Aug18.pdf.
11. Barreto SG. Editing for language: content and avoiding ambiguity in data presentation. In: Parija SC, Kate V, editors. Thesis writing for master's and PhD program. 1st ed. Singapore: Springer Nature; 2018. p. 199–205.

Checklist for Grant Proposal: Mandatory Elements

14

Medha Rajappa

For every minute spent in organizing, an hour is earned

Benjamin Franklin

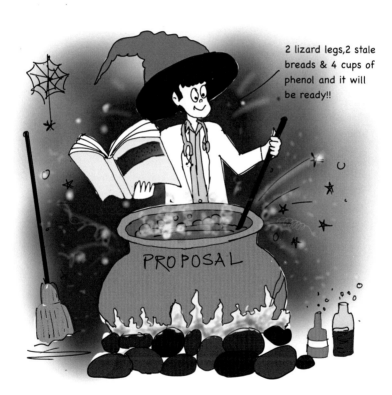

Checklist for grant proposal-mandatory elements

M. Rajappa (✉)
Department of Biochemistry, Jawaharlal Institute of Postgraduate Medical Education and Research (JIPMER), Pondicherry, India

161

S. C. Parija, V. Kate (eds.), *Grant writing for medical and healthcare professionals*, https://doi.org/10.1007/978-981-19-7018-4_14

Objectives
- To list the essential elements of the checklist for grant writing.
- To understand the requirements for successful grant writing.

This chapter deals with the essential elements of the grant application checklist, based on the guidelines available in various grant agencies [1–6] to get you a successful grant award. A checklist (Table 14.1) is provided at the end of the chapter, which lists these key elements and will be very useful for investigators who want to be successful in the award of grants. These suggestions are only a lead for you to understand this process, and the investigator is advised to familiarize yourself with the funding agency guidelines for their specific grant application process and ensuring compliance with the guidelines of the funding agency is most vital for the success of grant award.

Table 14.1 Checklist for grant proposal—mandatory elements

S. no.	Items	Yes/no
1	Novel ideas important in the context of the health needs of the country	
2	Grant idea driven by a strong hypothesis	
3	Logical rationale for project hypothesis	
4	Proposal fits with local, regional, and national priorities with relevant public health impact	
5	Work plan and methodology adequate to prove the project hypothesis	
6	Timelines and budget realistic and adequate to answer the research question	
7	Clear and concise, neat and well-organized proposal, with all headings filled-in with adherence to template and word counts as per the latest guidelines of funding agency	
8	Diagrams, graphical summary, flow charts, and concept maps to add clarity and visual appeal	
9	Multidisciplinary team with the expertise to carry out the work plan	
10	Adequate documentation for necessary approvals (IEC/IAEC/IBSC) and MOUs delineating the roles and responsibilities of each institution in the project	
11	Language, spelling, and grammar check for the grant proposal with font type and size as per the guidelines given	
12	Preliminary data from pilot studies to support the idea under consideration	
13	Linking of individual objectives, methods, and project outcomes to provide more clarity on the research question under consideration for funding	
14	Review of literature adequate to show the lacunae in the existing body of work	
15	Citations as per the required format of the funding agency guidelines	
16	Adequate time (at least 3–6 months) for planning, writing, reviewing, and revising the grant proposal	
17	Biographies of investigator team with adequate details regarding training, expertise, ability to lead a team, details of ongoing and completed funded grants and publication details from the last 5 years relevant to the proposed work	

14.1   Essential Elements for Grant Writing Application

Every grant starts with a seed, an idea that has germinated in the mind of the Principal Investigator. This idea should be novel, doable, and considered important in the context of the health needs of the country. So first, work on the idea and try to write a concept note which conveys the idea concisely, with all the required headings filled in as per agency guidelines. Contact the Program Officer of the agency (if allowed) and get feedback on the idea, your queries, and the funding opportunity in the agency to which you intend to submit the grant. Check the existing literature in your interest to check if the idea is novel. Ensure that your grant idea is driven by a strong hypothesis and that you are able to define what you are setting out to establish. Provide a logical rationale for your hypothesis. Explain how the proposal fits with local, regional, and national priorities and ensure that its public health impact is laid down clearly to the reviewers of the project. Ensure that your methods are adequate to prove your hypothesis. Ensure that the timelines and the resources requested are adequate to answer your research question. In short, the proposed initiative should be considered novel and doable. Those are the keywords to be kept in mind during grant writing.

Next, follow all the guidelines given by the funding agency on their website and ensure that you get ready a clear and concise, neat, well-organized, and visually appealing proposal, with all headings filled in as per the guidelines. Make bullet points, diagrams, graphical summary, flow charts, and concept maps to convey your idea to the grant agency and to sell your idea as doable and contextual in the background of the health priority needs of your country. Ensure a realistic grant work plan, timeline, and budget for the project. Set up a multidisciplinary team with the expertise to carry out the work plan, and this could be inter-institutional or from your own institution, depending on your project needs. Ensure that the adequate documentation for roles and responsibilities of each institution is well delineated in the final draft. Ensure that a preliminary review of the project is done by an expert team from your own institution or collaborators, whose suggestions can be used for the betterment of the project plan. Ensure that you check the websites of the funding agencies on a regular basis to get an idea of the latest funding opportunities and call for proposals that the agency funds based on the health priorities and needs of the community in the country. Depending on the specific research idea, it is good to get the documentation required, such as the approval of the Research Advisory Committee, Institutional Ethics Committee for human/animal research/Institute Biosafety Committee (as applicable) in place before the grant application is filed.

The language used in grant writing should be simple, concise, logical, and crystal clear. Check the agency website for the latest guidelines for the grant application. Ensure you follow the exact format given in the template in the grant guidelines. Word limits, font styles, font sizes, and margins as specified in the template in the grant guidelines should be complied with. Ensure that a language, spelling, and grammar check is done for the grant proposal. Print and review the application for appeal and for correcting errors, if any.

14.2   Tips for Key Elements of a Successful Grant Proposal Application

The title of the project should be concise, reflective of the proposed work, and create a favorable impression when reviewers read the proposal. The cover letter and project summary should be well written and self-explanatory. It should be easy for the reviewer to understand the felt need, objectives, and novelty of the project. Explain in clear terms why the idea should be funded and how it will add to the existing knowledge in the field. A review of literature should be adequate to show the lacunae in the existing body of work and how this idea will address the gaps in the published literature. If available, please provide preliminary data from pilot studies to support the idea under consideration. Explain how this can be expanded and translated into the larger grant project proposal. Stating the project outcomes and linking the objectives, methods, and project outcomes help reviewers to get a clear idea about the proposal at hand under consideration for funding. Also, outlining alternate methods which would be used to address the research question in case of potential problems gives a favorable impact on the reviewers. Discussing the statistical approach for data analysis and having a statistical expert on board is always useful while writing up a proposal. Ensure the budget is apt to address the objectives and the experiments for the project. Ensure that the timelines are really addressing the research idea at hand under consideration for funding. Ensure that the bibliography and citations are as per the required format of the funding agency guidelines. Try to avoid writing the proposal at the last minute. Ensure adequate time (at least 3–6 months) for planning, writing, reviewing, and revising the grant proposal before submission to the agency. Ensure you provide adequate details in your grant proposal about your investigator team regarding their training, expertise, ability to lead a team, details of ongoing and completed funded grants, and publication details from the last 5 years, which should be relevant to the proposed work. Early Career investigators should provide their biographical sketch and show that they have adequate institutional support and resources to carry out the project successfully. It is also imperative that the young investigators have collaborators for specific expertise and resources needed for the project. Having a mentor for guidance early on in their career for grant writing and project implementation is helpful for young investigators.

Lastly, if you face rejection the first time, use it as a learning experience and a stepping stone for success on the second attempt. Address the critique and reviewer comments with an open mind and invite subject experts to brainstorm how to address the issues raised, which led to rejection. Work on the proposal systematically and try once more the next time round, and success will be yours for sure.

14.3   Conclusion

To conclude, this chapter has briefed researchers about the main components of the grant proposal checklist. A word of caution is in order here. This checklist can, at best, be used as a preliminary guide to familiarize with the grant writing process, and it is mandatory for the researcher to check out the grant agency guidelines and comply with them for success of grant writing.

Grant writing is a painstaking, time-consuming, systematic process, with no guarantee of success to everyone alike, the first timer or the experienced doyen. Every time you start with a new idea, the same process is to be done meticulously all over again. Work on the idea, pen it down as a grant proposal and toil day and night, till it is ready. Perseverance is the key to success in grant writing. Wishing you all the best for your success!

Case Scenarios
1. A researcher is working on submitting a research proposal for monetary support to the funding agency. Which of the following are absolutely essential for the researcher's success of funding?
   (a) Novelty of grant idea relevant to emerging health needs of the country.
   (b) Methodology sufficient to provide answers to the objectives.
   (c) Pilot data available in support of the idea.
   (d) Sufficient expertise in the investigator team to ensure success of the study.
   (e) Approvals from necessary agencies for carrying out the study.
2. Can you list the essential elements of a grant proposal checklist?

References

1. https://www.wpi.edu/sites/default/files/inline-image/Offices/Sponsored-Programs/General%20 Grant%20Proposal%20Checklist5.2.16.pdf.
2. https://www.unco.edu/research/pdf/grant-writing-websites-docs/developing-and-writing-proposals/checklist.pdf.
3. https://mffh.org/wp-content/uploads/2016/04/Grant-Proposal-Checklist-MoCAP.pdf.
4. https://epms.icmr.org.in/extramuralstaticweb/pdf/Adhoc/1.ICMR_Guidelines_Extramural_ Research_Program.pdf.
5. https://www.serbonline.in/SERB/emr?HomePage=New.
6. https://dbtindia.gov.in/sites/default/files/Proforma_R%26Dnew.pdf.

Tips for Improvising the Chance of Getting the Grant

15

Rajesh Nachiappa Ganesh

Improvement begins with 'I'

Arnold H Glasow

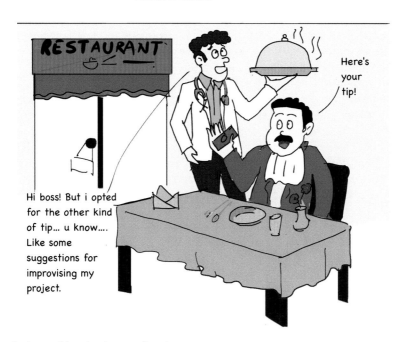

Tips for improvising the chances of getting a grant

R. Nachiappa Ganesh (✉)

Department of Pathology, Jawaharlal Institute of Postgraduate Medical Education and Research (JIPMER), Pondicherry, India

S. C. Parija, V. Kate (eds.), *Grant writing for medical and healthcare professionals*,
https://doi.org/10.1007/978-981-19-7018-4_15

Objectives
- Utilise the various tips for increasing the chance of grant proposal acceptance.
- Gain the perspectives of both the investigator and reviewer of the grant application.

15.1   Introduction

An application for a research grant is made with lots of expectations and many a time in a desperate attempt to enable the investigator to pursue their research ideas by the creation of facilities and providing funding to carry forward advanced work in their field [1].

Availing a research grant from a reputed scientific organisation is also a stamp of validation of the investigator's work in their chosen area of work. In addition to being a measure of the quality of the research work, a research grant attracts more research students and Ph.D. scholars, as well as helps in chances for collaborative studies. Above all, research grants provide an opportunity for developing expertise and increase exposure in the field of work for the investigator and help to train students and scholars in the latest scientific advances [2].

Thus, undoubtedly research grants open valuable opportunities and are sought by a large number of researchers. Every single grant call receives a very large number of applications and the chances of being shortlisted for extramural funding is not an easy task. In this context, we need to ensure certain basic rules are followed to increase our chances of success. First and foremost, the researcher should demonstrate and ensure clear focus in their field of work. A researcher who shows the continuity of research thoughts and ideas to address research questions in a particular area of interest is valued and stands a much higher chance for peer review [3].

15.2   Focus Your Area of Research Work

A professional committed to pursuing an academic career with an aim to build an atmosphere of research, and train Ph.D. scholars and post-doctoral students must learn to focus their work on an area that inspires them, from an early stage. Being a focused professional can be a daunting task in a country such as India, where most healthcare settings are highly crowded and multi-tasking is a pre-requisite and an essential requirement. In spite of all the compulsions and necessities in day-to-day patient care and teaching assignments, doctors, and academicians must be focused on their area of research pursuit. This ensures that the researcher is updated and gains greater levels of expertise and intuitiveness in their focused field of work. Most important, focused learning and consistent work in a field, enable the researcher to understand the limitations of scientific evidence and the need to find answers to research questions that will make an impact on patients and the community at large.

15.3 Continuity of Research Questions

Continuity of research ideas and the professional quest is an offshoot of a focused area of research. This enables a researcher to have command over their research work due to regular work experience in the field. In addition, a researcher will be able to demonstrate publications in the related field in which funding is being sought. To put it the other way around, a funding agency will have significant confidence in the investigator who demonstrates focused work with the continuity of research questions, as they are assured of good quality work and publications arising out of the funded project.

15.4 Clarity of Research Hypothesis and Innovative Thought

The investigator must be aware of the fact that most of the project proposals are scrutinised by experts from different domains and not by professional experts from the same field as the investigator. Hence, it is important to make sure that the research title and hypothesis are simple and clear enough for scientific scrutiny by a multi-disciplinary expert team. At the same time, a researcher should demonstrate innovative and effective solutions to the research question or hypothesis being studied. Another common error is the submission of a research proposal to establish a facility for patient care service in a hospital or healthcare setting. Investigators must be clear that research funding is exclusively meant for research ideas or questions which are presently unanswered and need research work to find solutions to the question. While a research idea that has potential translational value is rated higher, a proposal that tries to establish a facility for delivery of an already proven standard of care is unlikely to be successful, as it does not satisfy the innovation criteria for research funding.

The investigator must learn to position themselves as reviewers to assess whether their proposal evokes sufficient interest and is exciting to a broader audience, beyond their domain of professional expertise. The research proposal should be coherent and shows a clear thought flow in the execution plan to answer the research question.

15.5 Title of the Proposal

Most proposals are scrutinised and shortlisted at the level of title and the broad concept document. Hence a title that clearly highlights the research question and the broad research methodology gives the advantage to the proposal. Ensuring that the title follows a standard methodology such as PICO or PICOT format to answer "Population, intervention, comparison, outcomes and time" is one of the established tools to frame a good title. The investigator must ensure adequate time and thought is spent on the title of the study and broad concept document, as only those proposals which find merit on initial analysis at this level stand a chance for further review and scrutiny for funding [3, 4].

15.6   Focus on Research Methodology and Multi-disciplinary Work

Investigators must spend considerable time and sufficient reading to ensure that the research methodology chosen is scientifically robust enough to answer the research question satisfactorily. The investigator must demonstrate sufficient experience and expertise. This can be a challenge while answering a novel research question, as there will be a need for expertise from a wide range of professionals. The solution to this challenge is by enrolling co-investigators from different disciplines, as required in the methodology. This ensures that the experts in the funding agency gain confidence in the feasibility of meeting the research objectives. Also, the investigators must clearly demonstrate that the research proposal does not require overwhelming effort beyond their usual professional work and that the objectives are achievable in the proposed time frame [4, 5].

The research methodology must clearly define the objectives, scientific parameters to be studied, and a well-defined statistical methodology to evaluate the results. The investigators must also verify that their methodology is ethically acceptable and fulfils the national and international regulations for ethical research. The investigators must clearly state that informed ethical consent will be obtained from the participants and Institutional scientific and ethical approvals will be obtained from respective bodies. This is all the more important in multi-centre studies involving several institutions, as such approvals would be required from each institute and must be stated so explicitly in the proposal.

15.7   Clarity of Language

The investigator must plan their proposal in such a way that the language used is simple and explicit, even to experts from different fields. Avoiding complex jargon in the proposals and using clear-cut definitions and internationally accepted published guidelines for defining research parameters and outcomes helps in simplifying as well as strengthening the research document [4, 5].

15.8   Read the Guidelines for Grant Application

Being familiar with the guidelines of the funding application and being well prepared beforehand is an important prerequisite. Each funding agency is likely to ask for particular documents or information, and it will not be possible to collect all the necessary information at short notice after the call for proposals has been announced.

In addition, be on the lookout for funding opportunities that focus on specific target diseases or investigators who are at the early stages of their career, within a certain age range, etc. It is important to utilise such opportunities, as it will help the investigators to make a beginning in their research pursuit and successful completion helps them to compete for larger funding opportunities subsequently.

Once you have taken an effort and improved your proposal, it is time for fine-tuning your proposal to make sure that it stands out among thousands of others. This is possible by ensuring that you focus on the proposal from a reviewer's angle and critically self-analyse and review your own proposal.

15.9   Being Aware of the Larger Picture from the Angle of an Investigator

Get your timing right – Is your research question, in focus for the funding agency or in national or international priority?

Form an interdisciplinary team early with the required expertise to answer the research questions and the proposed methodology

Get your ideas vetted by discussing your proposals with senior colleagues in your area of expertise as well from your multi-disciplinary team

Assess your organization's resources. Frame your proposal according to the strength of the work in your organization and the infrastructure available

Review funding announcements and guide notices. Try and discuss your ideas with your research team to strengthen the proposal and make sure that the idea is conveyed clearly in the proposal

Be aware of your competition and the fact that your application must stand out among thousands of others

Have clear timelines. Be prepared beforehand with a detailed proposal and set timelines to achieve study objectives

Have clearly defined strategies and research proposal ready before the funding announcement

The broader strategy for evolving a successful strategy to get funds is depicted in a flow chart.

Get your ideas vetted by discussing your proposals with senior colleagues in your area of expertise as well from your multi-disciplinary team.

The major considerations that impact a reviewer when assessing a proposal are the title of the study and the concept note. The single most important point is the impact and novelty of the study proposal. Let us see this in a pictorial format.

15.10 Reviewer's Angle

Impact and Novelty – On a scale of 1 to 10

Is the study idea meritorious?

The novelty of the proposed work? Are the idea and the solution really novel?

What is the potential impact of the research work based on its potential results and translation value?

15.11 Fundamentals on Framing the Research Proposal

Developing a strong hypothesis/research question is the most critical and important step in the research proposal.

Is the hypothesis and/or research question valid and the level of evidence supporting it? Are the present lacunae in scientific evidence clearly spelled out in the proposal?

Is the methodology well designed? Have the investigators provided detailed procedures for the methods proposed in the study?

Have the investigators spelled out the aims and objectives in a clear and logical way?

Is the work environment conducive to the conduct of the research study?

Are the investigators qualified and/or experience to pursue the work in the field of work proposed?

The hypothesis should be strong and important to the proposed field of work. Investigators should ensure that the question/hypothesis is testable and will stand scientific scrutiny. There must be sound scientific rationale and critical thinking in the proposed hypothesis. There must be clarity on whether the investigators have evaluated alternate hypotheses for the problem and the strength of the proposed hypothesis. The most important pitfalls in the research hypothesis are that investigators must try to avoid a "fishing expedition" where the hypothesis is not a method in search of a research problem in the field of work.

15.12 Critical Steps in Preparation of Funding Proposal

Investigators must identify relevant and potential funding agencies that are likely to fund their field of work. This is achieved by thorough research of the various focus programs of the funding agency. It is useful to see their websites for previously funded proposals to get an idea of the focus of the funding agency. Investigators must be very self-critical and write responsive proposals and must have a genuine willingness to get feedback from peers [4, 5].

15.13 Research Proposal is Written for the Audience

Always critically self-review your proposal to ensure that the research question/ hypothesis and methodology are appealing and clear to a neutral scientific expert and inspire them to value the scientific merit in the work. The investigators must ensure that their writing is addressed to a general audience and it is a critical requirement.

15.14 Concept Proposal Development

Read widely in literature to grasp the existing scientific evidence and identify the lacunae and write your idea in a single page document to ensure that the needs are spelled out explicitly. Build your proposal document from your area of strength and expertise. Subsequently add experiments and interventions from other areas, where professional help is required by identifying partners from different specialisations to ensure that the work is feasible and can be completed professionally. It is sensible to build a team of co-investigators so that the research pursuits can expand together. Investigators must be open to critical inputs from all the team members, and peers and most importantly, be willing to self-review the document.

Once the idea is concrete, the investigators must ensure that the document is prepared exactly as per the guidelines of the funding agency [4, 6].

15.15 Identification of Relevant Funding Agencies

Have a clear goal to find potential funding sources, and this is achieved by multiple sources such as liaisons with peers who have obtained funds from external agencies. Other major sources are exploring websites of reputed funding agencies and studying their funding program guidelines in detail. Attending conferences and other educational meetings can be opportunities to interact with senior colleagues and peers whose inputs can be vital in identifying relevant funding agencies in the field of work. The investigator must be inquisitive about how the other institutions and Universities get funds for their research in similar areas of research as the investigator [4].

15.16 Research the Funding Programs of the Agencies

Investigators must study the goals and determine the priorities of the funding program and the selection process. This is made significantly easier as most reputed funding agencies give clear details on their websites. Investigators must have clear ideas on the program priorities and see who has been funded earlier, what are the factors in the decision-making process, the methodology, and process of peer review, total funding provided by the funding agency, duration of awards, and success rates in the previous years. Investigators must clearly weigh all these factors before deciding to submit their proposal to a particular funding program.

Program officers and reviewers of your research proposals are potentially your peers in your field of work and regularly attend conferences and professional meetings in the focused field of work, being communicative, responsive, and innovative in your professional circle helps in learning and refining your research priorities.

15.17 Propose a Realistic Research Budget

Another foremost focus for the investigator is to be extremely careful about the budgeting that is proposed. The investigator must ensure that their research budget is realistic. They must take extra effort to do a meticulous calculation of all the expenditure that is likely to be incurred and get quotes from major vendors for all capital and consumable expenditure. The investigator must realise that they cannot build all the infrastructure that they seek with single funding. They must try to get the most critical requirements from the funding and gradually build their research capability. This is a major factor, once the proposal has cleared the initial scrutiny and concept proposal stage [5].

15.18 Excel in All Categories

The investigator must demonstrate sufficient expertise, have deep knowledge and commitment to the proposed work, and ensure that the proposal is realistically feasible in their setting without undue effort. Ensure that the work is innovative and answers relevant questions so that publishing the results will be feasible in good-quality journals.

15.19 Proposal Document

The investigators must ensure that the regulations of the funding agency are followed exactly and clearly state the benefits and significance of the study in the abstract. Ensure that the time schedule that is proposed is well thought out and describe the deliverables at each time frame. There must be a clear justification of your proposed budget expenditure.

The proposal document should be clear in the goal that is set to achieve. It is a good practice to complete the proposal writing at least 3 weeks in advance before the deadline date and get feedback from peers and colleagues from your research team as well as from other institutions. In addition, it is a good practice to seek critical thoughts from researchers from other fields and feedback from totally unrelated branches to identify how well the document communicates the research idea.

A good research proposal that is chosen for funding exemplifies innovation and seeks significant improvement in the scientific understanding in the field from the study. The proposal should be able to convey that it has the potential to achieve this target.

15.20 Most Important Tips on Successfully Getting Funding

The proposal document is not reviewed by peer reviewers from the same area of specialisation most of the time. The reviewers look for the bigger picture and broader ideas. Also, the reviewers have several times the proposals that they can fund and hence look for major errors or blunders in the proposal to ensure that they are able to reject many. Thus, research funding is more a question of elimination rather than selection. Having understood that it is methodology is essentially aimed at elimination, the investigators must be wary of the reasons for rejection of proposals and should ensure that their proposals stand out and are not rejected [1].

The major reasons for rejections are highly ambitious and unrealistic proposals with unfocused aims or limited aims with a lack of clear future direction. Lack of originality or new ideas or lack of compelling scientific rationale, incremental or low impact research, and the inability to demonstrate expertise or publications in the area of the submitted proposal are common reasons for rejection of a proposal [3].

Hence please ensure the focused area of research with emphasis on innovation and significant outcomes, be responsive to the program, and take utmost care in writing the proposal making sure to demonstrate the capability to accomplish objectives.

Funding agencies want to accomplish that the program priorities are met, and they do not want duplication of earlier work. They are primarily interested in finding areas where there are lacunae in scientific evidence in the priority area. Funding agencies also prioritise investigators who demonstrate the ability to complete their projects and objectives on time and who do not have any professional black marks in their field of work or in earlier funded projects.

15.21 Conclusion

In conclusion, the chances of successfully obtaining a research grant can be dealt with from two angles. In the first perspective, the investigator must have a clear focus of research interest and propose a research question which is novel, valid, and scientifically relevant and has potential translational value. The investigator must also be able to substantiate their experience, qualification, and knowledge with previous research work and publications in the relevant field. An intelligent decision would be to have a strong multi-disciplinary team of co-investigators. Being self-critical of the proposal and taking multiple inputs to strengthen the proposal are potential tools to improve the quality and thereby the chances of success for funding. The second perspective is to critically evaluate the research focus and national and/or international scientific priorities of the funding agency. Choosing the appropriate funding agency by fitting in our research question and focus with their priorities, and critically reviewing our eligibility to fulfil the requirements of the funder are critical tricks in successfully obtaining research grants.

Case Scenarios
1. A researcher wishes to apply for a research grant involving characterisation of molecular signatures in a particular type of acute myeloid leukemia. He is interested in studying novel molecular targets on which there is limited literature. He has identified a funding agency which has prioritised funding in the field of acute leukemia. The investigator has expertise in utilising molecular methods in his previous studies with publications in the field of head and neck carcinoma and viral carcinogenesis. However, the person does not have any previous published work in the field of haematology or acute myeloid leukaemia. What strategies would improve his chances of successfully competing for a grant?
   a. Involve co-investigators with extensive experience and work in the field of acute myeloid leukaemia.
   b. Apply for the grant as a single investigator since he has expertise in the methodology in spite of limited work in the field of interest, where funding is sought.
   c. Tweak the research question to incorporate the documented field of expertise of the investigator by studying viral markers in the aetio-pathogenesis.

    d. Drop his curiosity in the new proposal and focus for research funding in head and neck carcinoma.

2. In a study of epi-genetic modifications and molecular signatures in rectal carcinoma using next-generation sequencing, identify potential areas of challenges and constraints during the conduct of the study and analysis of the results. Devise innovative and feasible strategies to overcome these challenges and strengthen your proposal.

References

1. Sohn E. Secrets to writing a winning grant. Nature. 2020;577(7788):133–5.
2. Ardehali H. How to write a successful grant application and research paper. Circ Res. 2014;114 (8):1231–4.
3. Gemayel R, Martin SJ. Writing a successful fellowship or grant application. FEBS J. 2017;284 (22):3771–7.
4. Wiseman JT, Alavi K, Milner RJ. Grant writing 101. Clin Colon Rectal Surg. 2013;26(4): 228–31.
5. Zlowodzki M, Jönsson A, Kregor PJ, Bhandari M. How to write a grant proposal. Indian J Orthop. 2007;41(1):23–6.
6. Arthurs OJ. Think it through first: questions to consider in writing a successful grant application. Pediatr Radiol. 2014;44(12):1507–11.

Dealing with the Rejected Grant Proposal: Learning from the Mistakes

16

Mitwa Joshi, Prashant Joshi, and Julian A. Smith

> *Success is not final; failure is not fatal, it is the courage to continue that counts*
>
> *Winston Churchill*

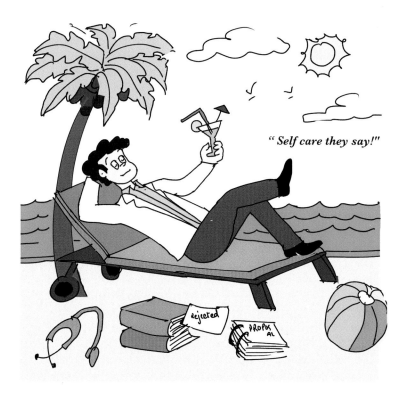

Dealing with rejected grant proposal-learning from mistakes

M. Joshi
Faculty of Medicine, Nursing and Health Sciences, Monash University, Clayton, VIC, Australia

179

S. C. Parija, V. Kate (eds.), *Grant writing for medical and healthcare professionals*, https://doi.org/10.1007/978-981-19-7018-4_16

Objectives
- To be familiar with where to search for feedback on a rejected grant proposal.
- To identify some of the common mistakes made when writing a grant proposal.
- To understand some of the strategies used to rectify issues in a grant proposal.
- To know where to search for alternative sources of funding.

16.1   Introduction

The process of having a grant application accepted by a funding organization can be quite challenging. This is due to a high degree of competition where funding organizations receive a high volume of applications, with only a small percentage receiving funding. According to Australian Research Council (ARC) data, the number of applications received by National Competitive Grants Program (NCGP) funding schemes from 2012 to 2020 was 57,352, with only 11,893 of these being successful in receiving funding—a 20.7% success rate [1]. In addition to this, data from the National Institutes of Health in the USA showed that their success rate for research grants was 20.5% in 2017 [2]. It is clear from this evidence that grant proposals are frequently rejected. The important steps moving forward from a rejected grant proposal are to recognize any mistakes made previously, attempt to revise such, and resubmit.

16.2   Sources of Feedback

Once a grant proposal has been rejected, it is crucial to forensically dissect the reasons for its knock-back. There are several places an applicant can seek feedback on their proposal.

An important first place is the funding organization that rejected the application itself. The rejection letter itself might contain some feedback or reasons for why the project was not funded. Deficiencies may be apparent upon reviewing any numerical score given to various parameters associated with applications under consideration. However, it may also be possible to ask for more feedback from the funding organization [3]. The comments may highlight some of the shortcomings of a proposal that can be amended for a greater chance of acceptance in future submissions. The feedback process can also aid in developing a relationship between an applicant and the funding organization as it demonstrates the applicant's dedication to a project. In some cases, funding agencies will lack the ability to provide extensive feedback on a proposal due to a lack of resources [3].

P. Joshi · J. A. Smith (✉)
Department of Surgery (School of Clinical Sciences at Monash Health), Monash University, Clayton, VIC, Australia

Department of Cardiothoracic Surgery, Monash Health, Clayton, VIC, Australia
e-mail: julian.smith@monash.edu

Supervisors, mentors and colleagues can provide invaluable support when it comes to dealing with a rejected grant proposal. They may have been in similar situations and can assess the quality of a proposal and appraise the feedback provided by the funding agency for its rejection [3].

16.2.1 Identifying and Rectifying Common Mistakes in Writing a Grant Proposal

16.2.1.1 Study and Research Methodology

Methodology

A study that aims to answer a research question with a poorly thought-out methodology is fundamentally flawed and will be unlikely to receive funding. It is important to cover different aspects of the study design and methodology thoroughly. Some of the factors that might require revising in a study could be:

- Grant assessors will require an applicant to adequately describe how they aim to collect data for their study. This includes the proposed equipment and processes to collect the data, the reliability of such, and how measurements will be standardized [4].
- Applicants need to explain how they intend to recruit participants for their study. This means a description of the factors that would include and exclude participants from a study, randomization methods, and whether participants were given incentives to take part in the study. If participants were given incentives, then there needs to be a description of the incentives and the possibility of these introducing bias into the study [4].
- A sample that is too focused on a particular group of individuals can seem too constricted to fund. This is because the funder will perceive the results of such a study as incapable of being generalized to a large enough population to justify the money invested [5].
- Poorly defined proposals are seen as too broad and therefore the aims are seen as being impossible to achieve. To mitigate this issue a participant can utilize the SMART (specific, measurable, attainable, realistic, time-bound) goals framework to better define their study's aim. In addition, the applicant should look to limit the number of aims as an excessive number can make a proposal appear over-ambitious and unrealistic. The aims of a study should also be independent of each other, meaning one of its aims should not rely on another aim being achieved [4].
- Failure to control confounders will mean that a study's results are skewed as there are now factors outside of the independent variable impacting the results. Managing confounders and an adequate description of how the applicant is going to do so is an important part of a grant proposal [4].

16.2.1.2 Preparing for Contingencies

Nailing the intricate details of a study is imperative in demonstrating an applicant's competency to see the project to completion. Despite this, those grading grant proposals are aware that there may be unexpected difficulties, barriers, and complications that can arise while conducting any study. However, a team that has a plan for if and when contingencies were to occur would appear to be far more favorable for funding [4].

16.2.1.3 Value of the Project

It is crucial that the study is perceived as having value to the funding agency. This can be through the study's ability to contribute to existing scientific evidence or the study's findings benefiting society [6]. Granting organizations will allocate greater funds to particular areas of study such as cancer and cardiovascular disease as new discoveries within these fields could yield large-scale humanitarian benefits. The National Health and Medical Research Council (NHMRC) allocated on average 116 million dollars towards grant proposals relating to cardiovascular disease from 2013 to 2020 whereas only 13.35 million dollars was allocated to grants which focused on skin disease through the same time period [7]. This is not to say that skin diseases are of less importance to society than cardiovascular disease, it is rather to highlight how grant-making organizations have priorities when it comes to what they believe are the most pertinent issues that need solving in the community.

Another way of thinking about the value of your project is to understand the economic outcomes that can be generated from the results. One area where this is particularly prevalent currently is when it comes to COVID-19-related research grants. Due to the large-scale economic outcomes that relate to the manufacture and distribution of the Pfizer COVID 19 vaccine, the company is providing grants for studies that explore the impact of efforts to overcome vaccine hesitancy [8]. This demonstrates that if a study aligns with the economic goals of a granting body it is far more likely to receive approval from the company as there is a potential return on the company's investment.

Even if the study is likely to yield evidence that will be of importance to society or contribute to scientific knowledge, this has to be evident within the proposal itself. This means that the proposal has to be written in a way that convinces the reader that the study has good reason to be supported.

16.2.1.4 Existing Knowledge

Another reason for grant application denial is that a granting body has already funded a project with a similar aim. The applicant should also be aware of any similar projects that have already been conducted or are in progress. When your research question is posed, it is important to carry out a literature review. This will assist in looking at the existing evidence and the quality of that evidence in order to judge whether the research question has already been answered [9]. It is also important to show the funder that you are aware of current knowledge and any knowledge gaps that exist within a particular field [4].

16.2.1.5 Pilot Studies

Carrying out a preliminary study can be useful in convincing a grant-making organization of your potential to conduct a large-scale project. Effective pilot studies will showcase how the major study has the potential to provide data leading to the confirmation of a given hypothesis [4]. A pilot study should be a demonstration of how a study's methodology has the potential to work rather than testing the hypothesis itself. The applicant should demonstrate how the study can work in a practical sense including information about participant recruitment, randomization, participant drop-outs, and other factors which will be relevant to the specific clinical study [10]. Including a pilot study and having quantitative evidence to support your proposal will boost the likelihood of having a successful funding outcome.

16.2.2 The Application

16.2.2.1 Alignment with Guidelines

Each grant-awarding organization will have its own specific set of guidelines that reflect an organization's intents. Therefore, it is crucial that a proposal matches these criteria. Guidelines, for example, might show that a granting body does not provide funding for scholarships, and this is likely grounds for rejection if this is what the applicant has requested [4]. The applicant should look to tailor their grant proposal to a single organization. A "one size fits all" strategy whereby the applicant submits the same proposal to various different funders is likely to fail as it does not demonstrate how your project is going to align with the values of the funder [6].

16.2.2.2 Formatting Issues

Incorrect formatting, structuring, and submission of grant proposals are all commonly made mistakes. However, they are easily amendable especially if the funder has clearly outlined how to carry out these tasks. If the funding body has provided instructions on how to submit the proposal, these details should be followed exactly as described [4]. If a detailed description is not evident, it may be useful to speak to a colleague or any individual with a previous grant application that was successfully funded by the organization. Reviewing a previously successful application can give the applicant an idea of the structure that is expected from the organization [11].

16.2.2.3 Budget Mistakes

When applying for a grant proposal, it is essential that the applicant sets out a clear outline for why a certain amount of funding is required and where these funds will be expended. One of the common mistakes in this section includes inefficient or overspending on unnecessary aspects of a project. An example of this could be overspending on human resources and salaries whereby the applicant could overestimate the number of staff required for a particular project which will increase the budget. By making cutbacks or finding efficiencies where possible an application can appear more appealing to a funder due to the lower costs associated with awarding such [12].

16.2.2.4 The Proposal was not Written Clearly and Persuasively

Frequently those reviewing grant applications will have read several other proposals. Therefore, writing an application that lacks clarity, organization, and explanations will diminish the hard work the applicant has put into formulating your study [13]. The applicant needs to have given himself enough time to organize the proposal in a manner that is logical. The aim is to write in a way that is pertinent and to avoid the use of filler words and jargon. Finally, it is absolutely essential to proofread the proposal, taking care to look for spelling and grammatical errors [13].

16.2.2.5 Timing

It takes time to craft a quality grant proposal so any applicant should look to leave plenty of time to prepare for some of the important elements, such as carrying out a literature review, gathering data from any pilot study, establishing the research team, and formulating a budget. It is reasonable to give yourself several months to even a year potentially to prepare a grant proposal (see Fig. 16.1; [11]).

16.2.2.6 Unrealistic Workload

A proposal that envisages an unrealistic amount of work for the research team is likely to be met with skepticism [14]. Occasionally, poor study design can be the reason for a study's workload being deemed unreasonable. Alternatively, it can be due to the way an applicant looks to manage their resources over time. One of the ways in which this issue can be overcome is by stretching the project out over a longer period of time. If this is not possible, the applicant might want to consider involving more collaborators in the project.

16.2.3 Issues with the Applicant or Team

16.2.3.1 An Inexperienced Applicant with a Poor Track Record

This is not necessarily a mistake but rather a shortcoming often experienced by applicants that do not have a large body of work and prior achievements to showcase to funding organizations. Funders are more likely to support grants from individual applicants or teams that have papers, awards, previous successful grant applications,

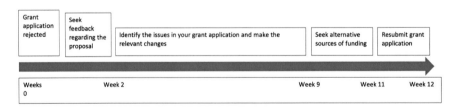

Fig. 16.1 A typical timeline of the steps following a grant application rejection. The duration of each of the steps will vary based on the quality of the initial grant proposal, the purpose of the grant proposal, and the reasons for rejection

and completed projects on their resumes. Experience with the specific equipment or methodology used in the study is also looked upon favorably when applying for funding. Applicants can collaborate with more experienced colleagues to assist with any aspects of a study for which they might encounter difficulties or lack experience. However, this does not mean that an applicant should involve an individual with an extensive publication history simply for the associated clout provided. Granting bodies will look upon this negatively if there are suspicions concerning this practice [11].

An applicant should engage an experienced team of collaborators as granting bodies look upon this favorably as long as all members listed are actively contributing to the project [9]. Having a good team of researchers is not only useful in convincing the granting body to support the proposal but it will also benefit the endeavor in the long run as they greatly facilitate the process of conducting the study.

16.2.3.2 Mistrust Between Funder and Applicants

Grant fraud is not a common occurrence especially when it comes to publicly funded grants. However, it still remains a concern for granting organizations [15]. For this reason, an applicant should look to assure funders that their money is going to be used appropriately. One of the ways this can be avoided is by carrying out and documenting a risk assessment in the application [12].

16.3 Seeking Alternative Sources of Funding

There are various different organizations, both publicly and privately funded, that offer grants to researchers. If your proposal has been rejected by a particular organization you may want to consider applying for a grant at a different organization once you have made the required adjustments to your proposal.

Examples of publicly funded research organizations include the National Institutes of Health (USA), the National Institute for Research (UK), and the National Health and Medical Research Council (Australia). Databases are a useful tool for applicants to find funding organizations and grant opportunities offered. GrantConnect is the Australian Government's system to streamline the identification of granting opportunities [16]. In the USA, grants.gov compiles a range of available federal grants [17].

There are also external, non-government organizations that provide funding for medical research. Specialty colleges such as the Australian and New Zealand College of Anaesthetists (ANZCA) [18] and the Royal Australasian College of Surgeons (RACS) both provide grants for junior and senior clinicians to conduct research within their area of expertise [19].

In addition to government sources of funding, private organizations may also be a suitable avenue to seek grants. The most effective way to explore this route is to become familiar with industry representatives or colleagues employed within the industry.

16.4   Conclusion

While it is reasonable for one to feel disappointed following the rejection of a grant application, it is crucial that the applicant does not give up hope. The process of writing a successful grant proposal is one that requires resilience and will require the input of senior colleagues and mentors. Overall, applicants should take the failure in their stride and strive to learn from past disappointments. An applicant should review their rejected proposal objectively, identify mistakes, and understand how to correct them for future submissions.

Case Scenarios

You are a senior resident interested in carrying out a large-scale retrospective cohort study. There is very little high-quality evidence that exists on your chosen research project. You have just had your grant application rejected by a major government-funding organization. You are not sure about the reason for the application's rejection because you believe the results from such a study would be beneficial to advancing the knowledge within your field.

a. What are two sources of feedback that can provide advice regarding the failed proposal?
b. What are three possible mistakes that could have occurred which led to rejection and how can each of these be rectified?

A surgical fellow has just had her first grant application rejected from a government-funding organization. The rejection letter highlights issues with the study including the applicant's poor track record when it comes to the field of research, the unrealistic workload for researchers associated with the project, and misalignment with the funding agency's guidelines. Despite her disappointment, the fellow looks to seek feedback from the funder as well as senior colleagues to see how she can improve the application.

a. Name the steps the candidate should go through in order to rectify the issues with the proposal.
b. What are three broad methods that can be used to rectify the issues listed above?
c. What are two potential alternative sources of funding the fellow can look to explore?

References

1. Australian Research Council. NCGP trends: success rate. 2020. https://www.arc.gov.au/grants-and-funding/apply-funding/grants-dataset/trend-visualisation/ncgp-trends-success-rates.
2. National Institutes of Health. Funding facts. 2018. https://report.nih.gov/fundingfacts/fundingfacts.aspx.
3. Crow J. What to do when your grant is rejected. Nature. 2020;578:477–9. https://doi.org/10.1038/d41586-020-00455-0.

4. Chung K, Shauver M. Fundamental principles of writing a successful grant proposal. J Hand Surg Am. 2008;33(4):566–72.
5. Grant Writing Mastery. Common reasons for rejected grant proposals. 2020. https://grantwritingmastery.com/common-reasons-for-rejected-grant-proposals/.
6. Indiana University-Purdue University Indianapolis. Some reasons proposals fail. 1998. https://www.montana.edu/research/osp/general/reasons.html.
7. National Health and Medical Research Council. Research funding statistics and data. 2020. https://www.nhmrc.gov.au/funding/data-research/research-funding-statistics-and-data.
8. Pfizer. COVID-19 Vaccine Grants. https://www.pfizer.com/purpose/independent-grants/covid-19-vaccine.
9. Zlowodzki M, Jönsson A, Kregor P, Bhandari M. How to write a grant proposal. Indian J Orthop. 2021;41(1):23–6.
10. National Institutes of Health. Pilot studies: common uses and misuses. 2021. https://www.nccih.nih.gov/grants/pilot-studies-common-uses-and-misuses.
11. Animate Your Science Team. What to do if your grant is rejected and how to ensure you get funded. 2020. https://www.animateyour.science/post/what-to-do-if-your-grant-is-rejected-and-how-to-ensure-you-get-funded.
12. Bellinger K. Top 10 reasons why grant proposals don't get funded... and how to improve your chances! 2015. https://www.linkedin.com/pulse/top-10-reasons-why-grant-proposals-dont-get-fundedand-bellinger-msw/.
13. Hume K, Giladi A, Chung K. Factors impacting successfully competing for research funding: an analysis of applications submitted to the Plastic Surgery Foundation. J Am Soc Plast Surg. 2014;134:59.
14. National Institute of Mental Health. Common Mistakes in Writing Applications. https://www.nimh.nih.gov/funding/grant-writing-and-application-process/common-mistakes-in-writing-applications.
15. Cayuse. Avoiding audit findings: examples of grant fraud and how to prevent it. https://cayuse.com/blog/avoiding-audit-recent-grant-fraud-cases/.
16. Grant Connect. https://www.grants.gov.au.
17. GRANTS.GOV. https://www.grants.gov.
18. Australian and New Zealand College of Anaesthetists and Faculty of Pain Medicine. Research Grants. 2021. https://www.anzca.edu.au/research/research-grants.
19. Smith J. Benefits of the Royal Australasian College of Surgeons Scholarship Program highlighted. ANZ J Surg. 2016;86:855. https://doi.org/10.1111/ans.13668.

Part III

Grant Writing for Specific Regional Funding Organizations

Preparing a Grant Proposal for Medical Research in the UK

17

Tae-kyung Park, Khaled Altarrah, and Rajive Mathew Jose

> *If I should die, think only this of me: that there is some corner of a foreign field that is forever England*
>
> *Rupert Brooke*

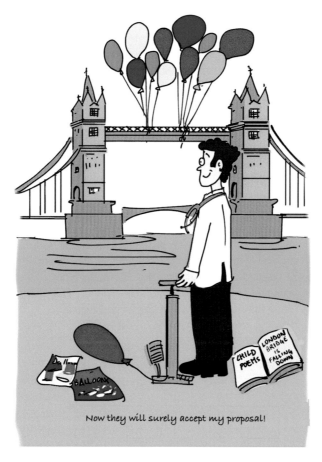

Preparing a grant proposal for UK

S. C. Parija, V. Kate (eds.), *Grant writing for medical and healthcare professionals*,
https://doi.org/10.1007/978-981-19-7018-4_17

Objectives
- To understand the sources of research funding in the UK.
- To understand the application process of research grants in the UK.
- To understand the role of the National Institute of Health Research (NIHR), the largest research funding body in the UK.
- To understand the assessment process for offering grants.
- Tips for writing a successful grant application.

Finding the money for research is not easy and the process of applying for grants can be tedious and often frustrating. There are several organizations that fund medical research in the UK. There are government organizations including charities, governmental bodies, pharmaceutical companies, and Royal colleges. The money offered through the grants from these bodies can vary from pump-priming grants of a few thousand to millions of pounds.

The grants applications for substantial funding are extremely competitive and a professionally written grant proposal is the key to securing them. While many of the established researchers with a reputed portfolio of research activities will be familiar with the application process, those who are starting their research career or someone who is doing research as part of their professional course may need some guidance as to how to write a successful grant application. The aim of this chapter is to give some guidance about the grant application process for medical research in the UK and give tips for a successful grant application.

17.1   Sources of Medical Research Grants in the UK

It is important to be knowledgeable about the various sources of funding for medical research in the UK. The Research and Development (R & D) Departments of Hospitals and Universities are often the best people to advise regarding the available grants and support you with the supplication process. There are several funding bodies that award research grants in the UK. The main types of funding bodies include UK Government organizations, research councils, and charities. Here are some examples of the funding sources that can be considered.

T.-k. Park
Medical Education, University Hospital Birmingham, Birmingham, UK

K. Altarrah
Faculty of Medicine, University of Birmingham, Birmingham, UK

Ibn Sina Specialist Hospital, Ministry of Health, Kuwait City, Kuwait

R. M. Jose (✉)
University Hospital Birmingham, Birmingham, UK

17.1.1 Government Organizations and Research Councils

17.1.1.1 Medical Research Council

Medical Research Council (MRC) is one of the nine UK Research and Innovation (UKRI) Councils to fund research. It was founded as a non-departmental government organization to distribute medical research funds in the UK. It was started in 1913 as Medical Research Committee and Advisory Council. Medical Research Council became under the Royal charter in 1920, and it has been instrumental in supporting many medical breakthroughs including the discovery of Penicillin. Medical research grants are advertised through their website (https://www.ukri.org/opportunity) and are awarded after a review by a panel of experts.

17.1.1.2 National Institute of Health Research (NIHR)

NIHR was founded in 2006 as part of the government's health research strategy, "Best Research for Best Health." It has been found that NHS Hospitals that have ongoing NIHR trials have a lower mortality rate [1]. NIHR funds a range of infrastructure for the NHS for research including the Clinical Research Network (CRN) and Biomedical Research Centres. They operate through several coordination centers across the UK. The funding opportunities through NIHR are advertised through their website (https://www.nihr.ac.uk/researchers/apply-for-funding/).

17.1.1.3 Innovate UK (Technology Strategy Board)

Innovate UK is one of the councils of UKRI that provides funding, supports, and connects innovative businesses for sustainable economic growth, including in biomedical research [2]. More information on applying for innovate UK funding can be found at https://www.ukri.org/councils/innovate-uk/.

17.1.2 Charities

17.1.2.1 Wellcome Trust

The Wellcome Trust was founded with legacies from Henry Wellcome a Pharmaceutical magnate in the UK in 1936 with the aim of funding research to improve human and animal health. It is the largest non-governmental research funding body in the UK and the fourth wealthiest charitable foundation in the world. They fund medical research in the UK and applications can be made through their website (https://wellcome.org/grant-funding).

17.1.2.2 Cancer Research, UK

Cancer Research is the world's largest independent cancer research charity and was founded in 2002 by the merger of two organizations, Imperial Cancer Research Fund and Cancer Research Campaign. It is funded entirely through public donations. Several notable anti-cancer drugs have been developed by scientists working with this organization. Applications for cancer research funding can be made through their website (https://www.cancerresearchuk.org/funding-for-researchers/applying-for-funding).

There are many trusts and foundations that provide grants in the UK. **Association of Medical Research Charities Directory** (http://www.armc.org.uk) provides a list of leading UK medical and health research charities, and **The British Academy** (http://www.thebritishacadmy.ac.uk)'s annual grant also supports the humanities and social sciences [2].

17.1.3 Pharmaceuticals and Industries

Several pharmaceutical companies and medical device companies fund medical research which is often in partnership with NHS Hospitals. Many of these are drug trials and these collaborations are done between the company and the R & D departments of the Hospitals or as part of a large multicenter trial run through larger research units. Research grants from industries for independent research are often advertised through their websites. If a researcher has a specific interest in a medical product and would like to conduct research on the topic, research collaboration is made through a contract between the company and the researcher's institution.

17.1.4 Royal Colleges

The Royal colleges of physicians and surgeons in the UK are the professional bodies for doctors and offer grants for research. Usually, they are small research grants such as pump-priming grants. These grants are advertised through their journals and websites.

The Royal Colleges provide training and development to medical personnel of various levels ranging from medical students to consultants. Hence, the Royal Colleges are integral organizations to the careers of medics and surgeons within the UK. Furthermore, one of the main objectives of Royal Colleges involves extending the frontiers of clinical practice and the development of novel treatments and techniques to enhance patient care. The Royal Colleges in the UK offer various research opportunities including grants and fellowships via an application process. Guidance and overview of the research application process of various Royal Colleges are available on their respective websites. It is important to note that Royal Colleges fund research related to their respective specialties.

17.1.5 Medical and Surgical Societies

Various UK medical and surgical societies offer to fund clinical or basic science research relevant to their respective specialties. Research opportunities via medical and surgical societies are not limited to medical doctors or surgeons, applications from allied disciplines are considered equally. Furthermore, various societies have designated committees and groups dedicated to research that can guide new researchers accordingly. Data related to the application process are located on the societies' websites. Furthermore, the society's secretariat can be approached for various queries and provide assistance when required.

17.2   Applying for Grants: Writing a Successful Application

Research grants are advertised through the websites of the relevant organizations. Some of the grants are offered for specific projects or topics whereas others are open to any research ideas. The format of the application varies between different organizations; therefore, it is vital to search for the right funding provider and read through their guidance before applying. Most organizations are now using electronic forms for submissions and some of them have tracker facilities that allow you to view the progress of your application.

17.2.1 Preparation

Writing a grant application is a major undertaking and can be daunting to new researchers. Firstly, the process to secure funding is fiercely competitive. Additionally, many funders do not accept resubmissions. Hence, it is imperative to prepare punctually and submit a solid proposal the first time around.

A good starting point when preparing grant applications involves studying the funding source. Performing a search of available grants and assessing the types of projects financed by various funding bodies can help identify the funder's interests. Funders offer grants based on study type (i.e., basic science or clinical) and perceived outcomes (i.e., biomarker identification, clinical practice modification, or social/epidemiological change) in accordance with the organization's mission. Once suitable funding bodies are identified, it is important to check assessment and eligibility criteria, as well as be familiar with their guidelines. Ensuring that the project, research institutions, and investigators meet the criterion can save significant effort and time. Furthermore, being aware of the general format and specific requirements of the application is important. Failure to comply with the criterion and guidelines can lead to application rejection at the first stage of the funder review process. Additional steps prior to application submission involve the identification and completion of any pre-submission registration requirements and developing a feasible and realistic timeframe to draft and revise the proposal, as well as making sure that it meets the application deadlines.

17.2.2 Proposal Content and Pitching

The ideal proposal should be concise, clear, and direct. It should be written in plain English to the funding body with the purpose of persuading the panel to provide the applicant with the required support. In such circumstances, it is important to know the audience and put oneself in the place of the reviewer. During the drafting process, it is best to remember that the reviewers may not be experts or related to the applicant's research area. Ultimately, the applicant needs to demonstrate to the panel that the research plan is fully considered and significant enough to advance a valuable cause. Furthermore, the applicant is required to show that they are capable, diligent, and responsible to accomplish that plan.

To maximize the chances of securing the grant, the application needs to convey the research plan thoroughly. A good proposal will include the problem to be addressed, the current data about the problem, and the investigations needed with clearly stated aims and objectives. In addition, research design, methodology, and execution strategy, as well as data and sample collection, storage, and analysis must be outlined. Ethical considerations and procedures, as well as the investigators, collaborators, and user engagement or hierarchy should be highlighted. Discussing study limitations and potential difficulties comes highly recommended. All this should be documented clearly and formatted accordingly as per the funding organization's guidelines. The use of spacing, bold or italics highlights and headings, as well as illustrations can make proposals easier to read and follow. Spelling typos, grammatical errors, and exceeding word limits are basic deal-breakers as these can cast doubt on the applicant's ability to execute and supervise their research. Furthermore, it is advised to write the proposal with the intention of connecting with reviewers.

With numerous research organizations applying for grants, it is imperative for the applicant to pitch their respective proposal eloquently so that it becomes identifiable and connects with the reviewers. One useful technique is scientific storytelling. Framing the information into a compelling story with the use of narratives can make the proposal more interesting, understandable, and relatable to the reader. The applicant, by being the narrator, can be influential by utilizing narrative factors, such as scenes, events, journeys, and reasoning, as well as demonstrating emotion, passion, humility, and vulnerability. All of which, can make the proposal stand out compared to other applications and increase the likelihood of success.

Finally, applicants should not fear rejection. Experienced scientists with success-ful grant submissions have gone through the same processes with unsuccessful outcomes. By maintaining a positive attitude, one can learn to improve and fine-tune their research and respective proposals to obtain a successful result. One such method is studying previously successful and unsuccessful grant applications. These can be acquired from trusted colleagues, university libraries, and online databases. One such website is **Open Grants** (https://www.ogrants.org/), which encourages researchers to openly and freely share their grant proposals to aid early-career scientists.

In general, most grant applications consist of filling out an application form and submitting supporting documentation. The key steps in preparation for a grant application are as follows:

1. Check the grant providers' website and guidance.
2. Outline your research idea and the available resources.
3. Work out the cost of the research program.
4. Get approval from the University or R & D department.
5. Complete the application form and submit it along with the relevant documentation.

There are several universal tips for writing a successful grant application. These include preparing the application in advance, revising the drafts many times, getting help from an expert researcher, and having a good communication with the organization offering the grants. There are useful articles available online which give general information on preparing a grant application [3].

As there are several types of application processes for grants depending on the funding organization and size of the grant, an example of applying for NIHR which is the largest funding body in the UK is discussed in detail.

All the information required to decide on your application and to plan your application is available through the NIHR website (https://www.nihr.ac.uk/researchers).

The first step is to check if your project is eligible for funding through NIHR. They fund research into health, public health, social care, clinical evaluation, and translation and technology development. They also fund research that produces evidence that healthcare professionals and policymakers can use to make informed decisions about healthcare and new interventions. They do not fund basic research or work involving animals or animal tissue. The next step is to find out which scheme to apply as there are several programs including Efficacy and Mechanism Evaluation (EME), Evidence Synthesis (ES), and Research for Patient Benefit (RfPB).

NIHR offers support in developing the application through the Early Contact and Management Service. It is important to consider the research question which should be relevant and clearly stated. The research question must be relevant to the NHS and the public. It is also important to consider if the research question will be relevant by the time the study is complete and whether the same research is being conducted elsewhere.

It is important to check if the application will meet their assessment criteria. The general assessment criteria can be found through their website and include the burden of the problem in the health care, what the study would add to the existing knowledge, and the impact of the study findings on health care. Value for money and scientific rigor are also important considerations when considering the grant application. It is also important to involve the patients and public by getting their views. This could be through interviews and questionnaires or media.

One should consider the research methodology and take help to check if the research design is appropriate to answer the research question. There are Research Design centers as part of NIHR which has regional offices across the UK. They can help with designing the methodology and their contact details are available through the NIHR website.

Planning for the impact of the study is an important step while planning your application. The impact is defined as the benefit the research will make to the economy and the public. It is important to outline the impact plan in your application which should include engagement with the patients and the public.

If the research is carried out in the NHS, one needs to get approval from the regulatory authority. If the study is from England or Wales, one needs to contact Health Research Authority or Health and Care Research Wales (HCRW). Approval is sought through a one-step application process through the website of the Integrated Research Application System (IRAS). Apart from the data for Health Research Authority it also captures all the data required for other regulatory authorities such as Research Ethics Committee.

Once these steps are completed the application can be submitted online through the NIHR website.

17.3   Assessment of Grant Applications

The process of awarding grant applications is after an assessment process that varies between organizations. In general, they go through a process of remit and competitiveness check, peer/lay review/assessment by a panel, and notification. The individual commissioning process is chosen by the organization depending on its structure, size of funds, and the type of research.

The assessment panel may vary and, in many cases, consists of researchers, lay members of the public, and patients.

Some organizations use a single-stage application process. The first stage is a triage process where the applications are screened to check if they fall within the remit of the funding body and that they are competing to be considered. They are then sent for an external peer review. Following this, they are assessed by the internal panel of experts considering the external peer reviewer's comments and scored. The mean score is used to rank the applications and decisions made as to which applications are to be recommended for funding (Fig. 17.1).

Increasingly many organizations are using a two-stage process. For instance, the largest research funding body in the UK, NIHR changed to a two-stage process in 2015 for their Research for Patient Benefit (RfPB) program. In this process, applicants are invited to send an outline application initially. These outline applications are assessed by a panel and scored. Based on the ranking they are invited to submit a full application. The full applications are sent to an external panel for review. The internal panel reviews the applications after that and is scored based on the external peer review comments and their own assessments. The applications are scored and based on the mean scores ranked to decide on the grant applications (Fig. 17.2).

In a comparative study of the one-stage and two-stage processes, it was found that the two-stage application process has cost and efficiency savings and more flexibility for applicants [4].

Fig. 17.1 One-stage assessment of grant applications

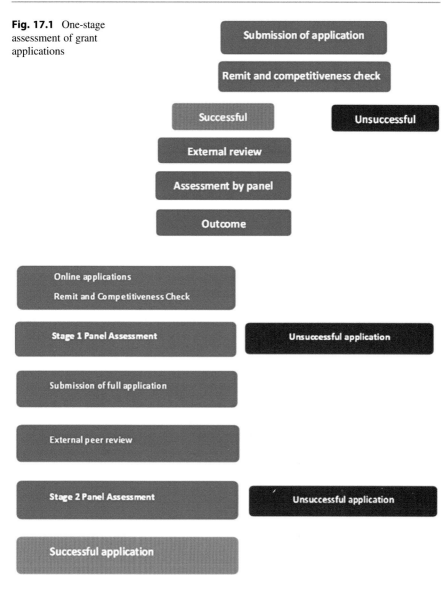

Fig. 17.2 Two-stage assessment of grant applications

Many other large funding organizations in the UK including the Wellcome Trust have moved to a two-stage process for simplicity [5].

There is increasing recognition globally that the grant application process is needlessly complex and time-consuming. An Australian study that conducted a survey amongst researchers found that a grant application took an average of 34 days per proposal and argued the case for streamlining and simplifying the process [6]. The two-stage process mentioned above seems overall more efficient by reducing the number of peer reviews and allowing more specific feedback to researchers.

17.4   Conclusion

There are several organizations which provide funding for research in the UK. These include governmental organizations, research councils, charities, and industries, Royal Colleges as well as medical and surgical societies. National Institute of Health Research (NIHR) is the largest funding body for research in the UK. Grant application is a structured process though the format varies between different funding bodies. Most of them are done now electronically with a provision to track the progress of the application. There are several tips for writing a successful application including preparing in advance, getting help from an expert and keeping a good communication with the funding body. The assessment of funding applications varies between organizations though they all go through a process of remit and competitiveness check, peer/lay review/assessment by a panel, and notification. Some organizations use a single-stage process though increasingly there is a move towards a two-stage process for application and assessment.

Case Scenario
Dr. RJ wishes to do a randomized controlled trial comparing two methods of metacarpal fracture fixations. He has written a research proposal and discussed it with the R & D department of his hospital who have agreed to be the principal sponsor for the study. However, there are several extra costs to conducting the study including the salary of a research hand therapist and the part-time salary of a research fellow. He decides to apply to NIHR for a research grant through the research for patient benefit (RfPB) grant offer. The R & D department helps with the preparation of the grant application, and he gets one of the senior researchers in the department to go through the completed application. The senior researcher suggests changes in the outcome measures as most of the measures are objective ones such as fracture healing times and non-union rates. He suggests including patient-reported outcome measures (PROMS) to make the study more in keeping with the RfPB ethos. As the study is conducted in the NHS, it required approval by Health Research Authority (HRA), and the application is made through Integrated Research Application System (IRAS). The application was submitted through the IRAS website and received approval from HRA and Research and Ethics Committee with minor recommendations.

The outline application is submitted and after stage 1 assessment he is invited to submit the full application. After 2 months, he gets the grant offer from NIHR. The hospital will receive the funds for conducting the trial and the study is ready for starting recruitment.

References

1. Jonker L, Fisher SJ. The correlation between National Health Service Trusts' clinical trial activity and both mortality rates and care quality commission ratings: a retrospective cross-sectional study. Public Health. 2018;157:1–6. https://doi.org/10.1016/j.puhe.2017.12.022.
2. NIHR Research Design Service London: how to find funding. https://www.rds-london.nihr.ac.uk/resources/how-to-find-funding/.
3. Arthurs OJ. Think it through first: questions to consider in writing a successful grant application. Pediatr Radiol. 2014;44(12):1507–11. https://doi.org/10.1007/s00247-014-3053-6.
4. Morgan B, Yu LM, Solomon T, Ziebland S. Assessing health research grant applications: a retrospective comparative review of a one-stage versus a two-stage application assessment process. PLoS One. 2020;15(3):e0230118. https://doi.org/10.1371/journal.pone.0230118.
5. Wilkinson E. Wellcome Trust to fund people not projects. Lancet. 2010;375:185–6.
6. Herbert DL, Barnett AG, Clarke P, et al. On the time spent preparing grant proposals: an observational study of Australian researchers. BMJ Open. 2013;3:e002800. https://doi.org/10.1136/bmjopen-2013-002800.

Preparing a Grant Proposal for the USA

18

Toishi Sharma and David J. Schneider

> *The world is a book & those who don't travel read only one page*
>
> *St. Augustine*

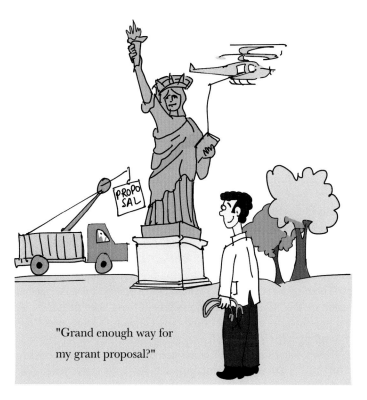

Preparing a grant proposal for USA

T. Sharma (✉) · D. J. Schneider
University of Vermont, Burlington, VT, USA

S. C. Parija, V. Kate (eds.), *Grant writing for medical and healthcare professionals*,
https://doi.org/10.1007/978-981-19-7018-4_18

203

Objectives
A focused preparation and appreciation of the review process can help to build a strong application, and therefore, the authors share general guidance and relevant tips to write an effective grant. The objective of this chapter is to assist the reader in developing a strong application by understanding:

1. How to plan effectively during the prewriting phase.
2. Essential elements of a grant proposal.
3. How to develop and write a winning-specific aims page and research plan.
4. Important basic principles that may be used in writing any grant application in the USA although the majority of them specifically pertain to the National Institutes of Health (NIH).

18.1   Prewriting Phase

It is a major undertaking to apply for an NIH biomedical research grant and a successful application requires ample time to plan, organize, and write an application that stands out and earns the funding to pursue scientific research [1]. The prewriting phase consists of understanding activity codes, identifying funding opportunities; reviewing the application requirements, and structure, effective communication with the NIH, pinning down the critical gap to develop a strong hypothesis, and identifying the research team and sites. These topics are discussed in detail below.

1. **Searching for funding opportunity announcements (FOAs)**: Although applications to NIH can be submitted by applying to generic funding announcements, researchers are encouraged to search for FOAs at Grants.gov, a portal used by all federal grant-making agencies including NIH. Each FOAs has a specific associated application form that must be utilized.
2. **Requests for applications (RFAs)**: The NIH invites proposals for research in defined areas with, generally, one submission date after which the invitation expires. These opportunities are particularly important because special funding is set aside by the NIH for awarding grants in these specified areas. All RFAs, past and present can be viewed in the NIH Guide for Grants and Contracts.
3. **Understanding activity codes**: The wide variety of research projects supported by the NIH are identified and differentiated by specific activity codes (e.g., R01, R44). An R01 is the standard independent research grant generally meant to provide 4–5 years of support for a project. It is important to note that certain NIH centers may not accept all types of grant applications or all activity codes and is therefore important to pay close attention to the FOAs to determine the participating NIH centers.
4. **Using NIH's RePORTER**: NIH offers a report expenditures and results tool which helps the researcher to search through an archive of NIH-funded projects and previous publications which can offer immense value in identifying the top projects funded in the specific area of interest by NIH, recognize other

successful grantees that may be associated with similar projects, and find expert collaborators for the proposed project. The relevant projects may be searched by utilizing specific terms or abstracts.

5. **Be mindful of the submission date**: The due date or application deadline is stated in the FOA. It is not difficult for the reviewers to identify when an application has been hurried and adequate time has not been allotted for proper preparation, budgeting, and overall presentation. Therefore, when in doubt, always consider submitting in the next cycle with adequate preparation. Start early to be able to complete the proposal and then give enough time for revision based on feedback from the research team and expert colleagues. This is particularly important because applications can only be resubmitted once. Even experts who have written multiple successful grants usually allot 1–2 months for feedback and revision.

6. **Criteria for prior approval from NIH**: Under certain circumstances, applicants may need to obtain approval from the NIH center at least 6 weeks before the anticipated submission date. For instance, when applying for a grant of over $500,000 for any year of the project. These approvals must be obtained well before grant submission and so require particular attention to the instructions and timeline.

7. **Applying for NIH grants from outside the USA**: Although the NIH grants funding to foreign institutions and applicants, the projects should be unique and should not be similar or equivalent to ongoing research in the USA for the project to be funded. Certain programs are not available to overseas nationals. Examples include center grants and Institutional National research service awards. To serve as a Principal Investigator (PI) on an NIH award, US citizenship is not mandatory. Factors favoring funding include the qualifications of the applicant as well as expertise and resources not available in the USA. It is highly recommended that an international applicant contact and regularly communicate with an NIH program officer throughout the planning and writing of the grant proposal. The contact information for NIH staff can be found readily on the internet.

8. **Pinning down the "critical gap"**: Reviewers consider numerous criteria for determination of scientific credit, and identification of the critical gap in knowledge that is intended to be bridged by the research is of utmost importance. It is the sole reason "why" research should be funded. The significance of the gap to be addressed should be clearly articulated. In this section, the question answered is "Despite the currently available literature and evidence, what is the critical barrier or knowledge gap preventing progress in a particular field or further optimization of patient care?" This section should be used to strengthen the application by clearly explaining the importance and significance of the gap and how bridging this gap will impact the field, treatments, or interventions in the future.

9. **Developing the hypothesis:** A successful grant tests a clearly articulated hypothesis. Developing a precise central hypothesis helps to demonstrate that

the research proposal is driven by current evidence serving as a starting point for further investigation to bridge the critical gap that has been identified.

10. **Innovation:** One of the key elements that drive the success of a grant proposal is addressing innovation because the NIH values research that aims to shift clinical and research paradigms. Innovation is not limited to technological aspects and can refer to a novel concept, methodology, unique multidisciplinary collaboration, or new intervention. Similarly, it may also refer to an innovative application of a well-established concept or methodology.

    Identifying the research team: It is important that all researchers and collaborators in the team have appropriate experience and training that will enable the team to successfully complete the project. For early-career investigators, reviewers look for appropriate mentors, and for established applicants, an ongoing record of advances in their field enhances the likelihood of success. In the case of multiple principal investigators, reviewers look for a good organizational structure that will work positively for the project. Ideally, the research team brings complementary strengths that will create synergy.

    (a) In general, the majority of research proposals require collaboration and partnership among different experts, and the NIH is committed to supporting such alliances. A research grant proposal with multiple principal investigators is often a strength of a proposal, particularly when multidisciplinary projects are undertaken, and a team approach is required. In these cases, expertise and leadership approach should be appropriate for the project, and a leadership plan should be included. Each collaborator will submit a letter of commitment which goes into the application and a separate letter to reflect the charge for consulting services.

    (b) It can be very useful to determine early in the process if one qualifies as a new investigator based on NIH rules. Special funding opportunities and awards are available to new investigators, and reviewers are instructed to give consideration to early career and new investigators. The criteria can be found on the NIH webpage. Although having a senior mentor is beneficial for early-career investigators, refrain from recruiting research personnel based solely on their "seniority" or position in the department who do not have a significant contribution to the proposal, as this will be readily apparent to reviewers.

11. **Selection of research sites:** A helpful means to identify the appropriate sites is to first have a good understanding of the resources needed to complete the research including staff, laboratory space, critical reagents, techniques or methods, equipment, and subjects for enrollment that are essential to the project and add innovation. Once these have been identified, conduct an organizational assessment to ascertain what resources are available and what additional support may be needed. Before including any site, ensure that it has adequate facilities as well as a conducive environment for research. Applicants should clearly state that they have the required resources for conducting the project and when possible include letters of commitment for these resources.

18.2 Writing Phase

An appointed panel of non-federal scientists reviews each application at NIH. Although the acceptance of any proposal depends on multiple factors, scientific merit holds significant weight. The reviewers assess each application with pre-established score criteria with a separate score for each criterion, additional review criteria, and an overall general score meant to describe the potential impact of the study. The knowledge of these criteria can greatly assist in writing a focused plan that appeals to the reviewers. These criteria are further elaborated in the research strategy section.

Researchers should follow page limits specified for each attachment in the grant application. Limitations vary depending on the application. Additionally, before writing, be sure to read the grant instructions and check specific instructions regarding the types and size of accepted fonts and specific formatting. Select appropriate spacing between lines so as not to make it overcrowded. Figures to explain important data or models are highly recommended but ensure optimal size, color, and fonts. Do not assume that reviewer will be able to expand the figures electronically to review them, and they should be easy to read and comprehend on a printed version. Refrain from using any abbreviations.

Know that there is no one style that is guaranteed to be successful, and writers have the flexibility to present their proposal in a way that they consider best. The written proposal consists of two major elements (1) Specific aims and (2) Research strategy. The research strategy can be further written down under three subsections addressing (a) scored criteria, (b) each aim in detail, and (c) potential pitfalls and limitations. We recommend the following sequential approach for writing the grant proposal.

18.2.1 Specific Aim/Aims

This component of the grant proposal will have the greatest impact on the success and so merits substantial time and effort. Reviewers usually have multiple grants to evaluate in a limited time frame, and therefore the specific aims page must capture the attention of the reviewer by conveying the important objectives in a careful and concise manner. It should begin with a succinct and sufficient background showcasing pertinent preliminary results that will allow the reviewer to understand the context of the proposed project.

The trick to writing an engaging background is to start by telling a good "story" and remain internally consistent throughout the proposal. Explain the critical gaps in knowledge and why is it so important to study them. The specific aims should test a hypothesis, develop a unique design, challenge current clinical practice, develop new technology, and address a barrier to progress in the field.

It is important to know that the reviewer may or may not be the expert in the specific niche, and therefore the key is to convey the objectives in simple terms, readable by a more general audience, highlighting the big picture rather than diving into excessive detail in this section. Experts recommend no more than two to three aims that are related but still independent. Avoid one aim being dependent on another because the failure of one aim would then doom the entire project.

Another recommendation by experts is to present the data, a novel concept, or a model through figures to make them simpler to understand and shorten review time, something that reviewers really appreciate. In addition to stating concise aims, describe how their completion will change the current clinical practice, technical capabilities, scientific knowledge, services, treatments, or interventions. Whenever applicable, novel theoretical concepts, methods, and interventions should be explicitly stated.

18.2.2 Research Strategy

18.2.2.1 Part A. Addressing the Scored Criteria

The reviewers assess each application with pre-established (1) scored criteria with a separate score for each criterion, (2) additional review criteria, and (3) an overall general score meant to describe the potential impact of the study. The knowledge of these criteria can greatly assist in writing a focused plan that appeals to the reviewers.

The scored criteria are as follows

1. *Significance of study*: Does this research address an impactful problem? Significance should be highlighted and central to the critical gap that is identified. Because the reviewer may not be an expert in the specific field of study, the importance of the gap must be clearly articulated and supported with literature references and preliminary results. An internal review of the proposal by someone who is not an expert in the specific field of study can be very helpful to ensure that the significance of the critical gap is clearly evident.

2. *Adequacy of investigators*: Do the members of the research team have the necessary training, background, experience, and credentials to conduct an effective study? All investigators are required to submit their bio-sketch, which gives them an excellent opportunity to add details about how their experience and expertise, either through training or publication record, make them a good fit for the project. Use the bio-sketch advantageously to identify three to four areas of science and link your related publications, if any, to prove why you are the appropriate person for this project and will be able to handle it efficiently. Demonstration of collaboration between team members enhances the likelihood of success of the application. The principal investigator should include a personal statement in her/his bio-sketch with enough evidence to demonstrate required training, experience as well as prior examples of leadership because reviewers understand that a project is likely to collapse in the absence of good leadership. For more details, refer to "identifying the research team" in the prewriting section of this chapter.

3. *Innovation*: Does the study include a novel theoretical or practical question? The innovation element can be one of the three types: conceptual, technical, or

collaborative innovation, depending on the project. These refer to a new idea or model, cutting-edge technology, or unique collaboration of researchers from different areas of science, respectively.

4. *Approach:* Is the research designed to achieve the stated goals? The reviewers are looking for an unbiased, robust approach. The ability to effectively address the hypothesis is a major driver of the overall impact score as it is meant to convince the reviewer that the project is practically feasible. For example, a study may have precise aims and all the available resources, thereby receiving the highest score possible in all the previous criteria; but if the approach receives a poor score, the grant is likely to be turned down.

5. *Environment:* Is the scientific environment conducive to the research?

Although not mandatory, we suggest addressing each of these five criteria as bullet points. This demonstrates key aspects of the project and assists the reviewer who must specifically comment on these aspects of the proposal.

The *additional review criteria* include appropriate steps taken to protect human subjects from harm; ensure appropriate inclusion of women and minorities, and details regarding handling biohazards and vertebrate animals, as applicable.

In the case of clinical research, adequate plans should be presented to include subjects from both sexes, and different ethnic groups and to avoid racial disparity. Plans to recruit subjects will be evaluated in great detail and therefore researchers should clearly state what measures will be taken; to protect human subjects from research risks; including minorities and other at-risk populations, as is justified regarding the research strategy proposed. The NIH inclusion of minorities' policy website has resources to determine which studies may be subject to NIH inclusion policy and should be reviewed by the applicant.

18.2.2.2 Part B: Addressing Each Aim in Detail

The research strategy should be written clearly to convince the reviewer that the specific aim is well-reasoned based on evidence in support (from literature and preliminary results) and that the proposed methodology is appropriate to achieve the specific aims. We suggest that each aim be described separately with (1) *brief background,* (2) *experimental design,* (3) *statistical analysis, and* (4) *anticipated results.* Begin by restating the aim before diving into the background specific to the aim. In the *experimental design,* list key details applicable to the study that will demonstrate the ability to complete the proposed studies.) Give appropriate references to your prior publications whenever possible to substantiate and add credibility to the proposed design.

For early-career investigators who may not have prior supportive publications, remember, NIH is looking to support them and therefore in such cases relies on appropriate collaboration with investigators who have demonstrated expertise in the field. Therefore, as previously stated in the research team section, it is important to involve the right people with the required knowledge that is pertinent to the research. This will give the reviewers assurance that the principal investigator will have appropriate support and guidance to complete the project and address unanticipated problems.

Incorporating a robust plan for *statistical analysis* under the guidance of an established statistician is an essential part of the research proposal. The inclusion of an expert in statistics as a co-investigator enhances the likelihood of success. This section should be well reasoned and aim to precisely identify the intended sample size, power of the study, data collection, storage, and statistical tests that will be used during the analysis.

The next section is *anticipated results*. This section will describe anticipated results and can be used to discuss how those results will bridge the critical gap and lead to future studies. This section emphasizes how the aim addresses the critical gap and maintains internal consistency within the proposal.

18.2.2.3 Part C: Potential Pitfalls and Limitations

It is crucially important to include a paragraph describing the potential pitfalls and limitations as well as strategies to address them. It indicates that the research methodology has been well thought through by the investigators and proposing alternative approaches indicates expertise and the ability to handle both anticipated and unanticipated problems. Use this section cleverly, showcasing the team's knowledge and problem-solving skills. Identify important and obvious limitations. Refrain from making it too long or identifying too many pitfalls, as doing so may negatively impact the proposal. Always end the limitations section on a high note.

18.3 Budgeting

This can take a substantial amount of time in the writing process and should not be delayed. The Funding Opportunity Announcements (FOAs) describe the type of budget required for the specific project. Developing a budget requires significant coordination among researchers, department lead administrators, and the central grants office.

18.4 General Instructions

A detailed data sharing plan, whenever applicable, should also be included in the application. Using URLs is prohibited by NIH to avoid large amounts of data in the application, diluting the topic, and adding load for the appointed reviewers. Although writing a successful application for NIH funding is a major undertaking, with timely planning, organization, and the right attitude, is it very doable. As Dr. Cipolla, recipient of multiple NIH grants states "Write a grant to get it, not to submit it."

18.5   Conclusion

A successful grant application requires ample time to plan, organize, and write an application. During the prewriting phase, authors should aim to understand different available grant codes, identify funding opportunities, effectively communicate with the NIH and pin down the critical gap to develop a strong hypothesis. The writing phase should focus on the predefined score criteria used by the reviewers to maximize chances of grant approval.

Case Scenario
Enumerate the items of the scored criteria for a grant application under the NIH

1. Significance of study
2. Adequacy of investigators
3. Innovation
4. Approach
5. Environment

Acknowledgements   Dr. David Warshaw Ph.D., for his expert contribution to the specific aims of section. Dr. Marilyn Cipolla Ph.D., for her expert contribution to the research strategy section. Dr. Mark Nelson Ph.D., for his expert contribution to the significance and innovation sections.

Reference

1. https://www.nih.gov/.

Preparing a Grant Proposal for Australia   19

Shubhum Joshi, Prashant Joshi, and Vaishali Londhe

Don't worry about the world coming to an end today. It is already tomorrow in Australia

Charles M. Schulz

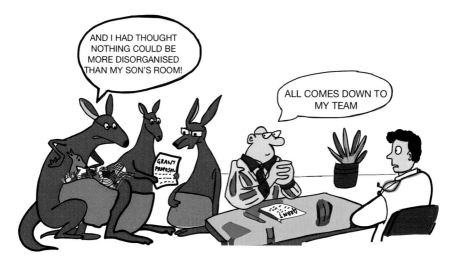

Preparing a grant proposal for Australia

S. Joshi
Wollongong Hospital, Wollongong, Australia

P. Joshi (✉)
Department of Surgery (School of Clinical Sciences at Monash Health), Monash University, Clayton, VIC, Australia

Department of Cardiothoracic Surgery, Monash Health, Clayton, VIC, Australia

V. Londhe
Department of Anaesthesia, Royal Victorian Eye and Ear Hospital, Melbourne, VIC, Australia

213

Objectives

- To understand grants and applications in Australia.
- How to conduct research into grants.
- To format and write an appropriate grant application for the different types of grants.

19.1   Grant Proposals

Australia provides many opportunities for medical research. The Australian Bureau of Statistics reports that from 2018 to 2019, government organizations spent a total of $3.3 billion on research and development projects [1]. Of this, healthcare-centered were awarded $726 million. There is a large amount of funding available for medical research projects in Australia, which would be available through these grants.

19.2   Sources of Funding in Australia

A grant proposal is a means to obtain funding for your project. It is a crucial step in much larger projects as the lack of adequate funding can render any potential investigation or publication void. This is especially true in laboratory-based research endeavors, multi-center studies, or prospective studies. As such, a grant proposal is the first step towards making sure your research meets its goals. However, there are no guarantees of getting funded. Dr. Carol Greider, the 2009 Nobel Prize Winner in Physiology or Medicine, had a grant proposal rejected the very same day that she found out she won the Nobel Prize for her discovery of the telomerase enzyme [2].

There are several sources of funding, each will have a different expectation in their grant proposals, but almost all of them will need a proposal. A major avenue for medical professionals in Australia is the National Health and Medical Research Council (NHMRC) which is run by the Australian Government. The funding provided by the NHMRC as part of the development grants for projects commencing in 2021 ranged from $634,492.20 to $1,107,069, with a total of $14,978,659.94 given towards medical research that year [3].

It is expected, however, that one should apply for several grants, expecting that not all of the proposals will be accepted. These include direct government funding and research institutions as well as private donors and companies.

19.3   Grant Applications

When applying for grants, it would be helpful to understand the general process behind a grant proposal being accepted. In general, a grant proposal is presented to a council within an organization that will review every relevant proposal. The council will then decide on the distribution of their budget for all the accepted projects.

As an example, project proposals submitted to the NHNRC are peer-reviewed by experts in the relevant fields who will then give their opinion on which projects should be funded. Smaller funds will be less likely to involve experts. This is important because the use of language will change when directing a proposal to experts within a specific field compared to people who may not possess that knowledge.

Most of the time, the proposals are reviewed by a board that looks through every appropriate application and discusses the merits of each one. For the NHNRC applications, the committee consists of experts from that particular field of biomedical science and submit reports based on what projects believe should be funded and which ones are unlikely to produce tangible results. Depending on the budget allocated, these projects may go through several rounds of reviews, with the committee members often asking for more information from the applicants to provide more evidence if a project is worthy of a financial grant.

Rejections are usually notified earlier, giving the applicants more time to re-budget or apply for other open grants. A rejection is unlikely to provide thorough feedback although some committees may state whether or not your project was within the guidelines of their grant. Usually, these rejections come out the earliest. Rejections that come later are more likely to have been discussed thoroughly but ultimately have lost out to other projects. This is usually where a better proposal would improve one's project's chance of being successful in obtaining a grant.

A successful grant would be allocated a particular amount of funding which would be given during that particular funding cycle.

19.4   Research the Grant

Before looking for grants, it is important to do an objective assessment of your own project. The main point is to identify costs, realistic deadlines, other funding avenues already available to you, and what you expect to achieve overall from your project. This will be important to mention in a proposal as projects with no clear or realistic goals and limited opportunities to obtain updates would be less likely to be accepted by any grant committee.

When researching grants, it is important to keep in mind that there are several different types of grants: research grants, educational grants, and personal grants. Research grants, as the name describes, are allocated to research projects. Educational grants are given to organizations or projects aimed at educating the community on a particular field or just in general. Educational grants are often community-based. Personal grants are given to individuals. This is often similar to a scholarship and is based on the individual's or organization's merits or situation rather than any particular project that is being undertaken. Some of these may be hardship grants aimed at someone struggling in some way. The individual or organization can choose to allocate the funding as they see fit.

If your organization has been deemed suitable to apply for a particular grant, it is crucial to perform extensive research on the grant as well as on your own project.

The first thing is to read up about the grant's specific application instructions, which vary from required supporting documents to expectations on updates and goals. Occasionally, these written proposals will be accompanied by a presentation or interview to further narrow down suitable candidates.

19.5 Commonly Requested Documents

Different organizations have different expectations when it comes to supporting documents. Commonly requested documents include cover letters, a curriculum vitae for project members, ethics approval reports, tax-related documents, and previous projects and their outcomes [3].

The next step is to learn about the organization behind the grant you are applying for. Different organizations will have different goals, and, as such, any written proposals to them need to target the specific aims of the organization [4]. This can be determined on their websites or by contacting the organization directly. In general, government-led grants would have slightly different goals and targets from a charity organization or a private company. Charity organizations should be approached using a more human-centered framework—how would the current project meet the aims of the organization and help their targeted population? For example, the Australian Institute of Aboriginal and Torres Strait Islander Studies (AIATSIS) would provide grants aimed at a variety of areas related to Aboriginal and Torres Strait Islander peoples, and a grant proposal to an organization such as this would need to discuss the impact of the project towards Aboriginal and Torres Strait Islander populations [5]. As a separate example, Pfizer is a pharmaceutical company that also provides grants for research projects [6]. The focus on a private company may be more about profit (although not always), and any grant proposal submitted to them should include any potential for the project to make money at some stage.

Another relevant is to find out the allocated funding the organization has. It is important, once any project's budget is determined, to apply for sufficient funding. A single organization may not fund the entirety of a project and often have a cap as to how much it will allocate to a single project at a particular time. Thus, in order to secure appropriate funding, it is important to know how many grants to apply for.

19.6 Abstract

Like any scientific publication, an abstract is a useful way to summarize the content of the proposal. This is more important in a grant submitted to major institutions, which would go through hundreds if not, thousands of applications. An abstract serves as a quick overview as to what the grant is about but also as a reminder to the grant committee as to what your proposal is about when reviewing applicants.

Unlike abstracts for scientific journals, this abstract will likely not have any results or conclusions. It just needs to include enough details about the area of study or project, the significance of the problem, and the aim of the project.

19.7 Introduction

The introduction to a grant proposal should be an introduction to the project itself. Like in any research paper, an introduction should identify an issue. However, unlike a journal article, the issue should be within the community or a medical problem rather than a gap in the literature. Once that has been briefly established, discuss the project you are proposing and how it aims to manage this particular issue [7]. The introduction should also briefly mention how your particular project is different from previous studies or projects.

An introduction needs to be short and to the point while simultaneously being "eye-catching." Its aim is to get the reader to be invested in the project and have an understanding of how it's relevant to their particular grant.

An example of how to start off the introduction could be by briefly introducing yourself. "My name is _____ and I am a researcher specialising in _____." This allows your proposal to have a more personalized approach. Another way is to introduce yourself as part of a research institution with a significant reputation "I am one of the researchers working in _____."

After introducing yourself, it is a good idea to mention the issue your project is working on. If this is a proposal to a government body, it will likely go-to experts in the field so you can be a bit more detailed or technical in your explanation: "_____ is a rising cause of morbidity in Australia, however, there is a lack of adequate techniques to effectively screen for _____ in our community." It is a good idea to reference your sources when speaking to experts.

For a grant not run by experts in the field, it would be best to simplify your explanations and the actual impact of the problem and a what your project aims to achieve: "_____ has been a been responsible for a large number of deaths or illness in Australia. Thus far there is no appropriate way to test for _____ but our project is looking for a viable way to do so which could benefit our communities by introducing early diagnosis or screening for risk factors." It is a good idea to keep technical jargon to a minimum and appeal to a more human-centric approach.

A private company would also involve experts to assist with decision-making. However, it will also be looked at by potential investors. As a result, there needs to be a balance between very detail-orientated explanations of the project and presenting the project as a good investment opportunity for the company. It is important to note that not all grants offered by private companies are allocated to projects for the sake of profit and organizations do offer charitable grants as well [8].

19.8   Discussing the Issue

The next segment should be aimed at elaborating the extent of the issue that your project is investigating. This is a good opportunity to build up to why your project is important and deserving of this grant. The paragraph, like the introduction, should be tailored to the recipient of the proposal.

When submitting the proposal, the issue needs to be clearly highlighted and its significance clearly explained. Like the introduction, a description of the issue needs to be modified depending on the audience of the proposal. For a grant from a community-based organization, it will depend on the organization, as to how much explanation is necessary. When applying for a grant from, for example, the Cancer Council, explanations of the impact of a particular type of cancer can be shorter as it can be assumed that the reader would have a basic understanding of this [8]. However, when applying for a more general grant, it is important to explain the area you are researching more thoroughly, especially if it is a niche area. An example of how to start is "_____ impacts at least 3 in 100 people annually and the prognosis of anyone diagnosed with it can range from 5 to 8 years. The financial impact of _____ is up to $200 million dollars a year." It is also important to discuss the pathophysiology briefly if your research deals with specific areas in dealing with the issues. For example, if researching particular genetic mutations in a disease, it is crucial to use simple languages to explain how the research relates to the disease and the potential for management or diagnosis your research brings to the field.

When submitting the proposal to experts, however, it is important to provide more detailed evidence to the grant committee. The amount of detail should be more than that presented to a non-expert. The idea is that the more detail with evidence to better convince the committee. A summary of the pathophysiology, targets, etc. of the disease should be outlined in order to show where your project aims to fill the gap in research and, subsequently, why it should be funded.

This concept is similar to a proposal submitted to a private company. If there is any evidence as to how the research could contribute to an economic impact on the company, it should be mentioned, but this is not always necessary.

19.9   Body

The body of the proposal should discuss the overall plan of this project. This is an explanation of what your project involves, the expected timeframe, and the results you aim to obtain. Basically, this paragraph exists to explain why your project needs the funding and the assurances you can provide that the funding will be used to further research or educational goals. Normally, the body is the largest segment of the proposal. The variability in this paragraph will depend on what the proposal requires which will vary from grant to grant. If the previous segment has discussed the issue, this segment is ideally where they will be elaborated further with evidence, previous publications, and what the project aims to accomplish regarding the issue.

When detailing the project for grant committees who are not experts, the body should outline briefly what your project involves and how it aims to resolve the issue that was previously discussed. Simple explanations with diagrams (if allowed) must be used. Include details of where the money will go (statisticians, tests, etc.) and the types of results your project will bring about. The writing style should appeal to both the logical side and a more sentimental description of the need to fund this project. However, the body should still include a simplified plan for the project in terms of expected results and timeframes. This may change depending on the requested formatting for the proposal.

A proposal submitted to experts needs to include more detail. The amount will depend on a word-count limit but should provide evidence that your project is scientifically viable, clinically or economically significant, and achievable in an appropriate timeframe. References to other publications should be included as well.

The methods would belong within the body section of this chapter. The description of the method should be brief. It is not the goal to be able to replicate the experiment but to make it clear to the reader that the project is following a scientifically sound process and will demonstrate the necessary results. Ideally, the methods should suggest where the cost of the project would arise from and provide evidence as to why this particular research project needs funding—biochemical testing, participants.

It is also useful to include previous studies related to this particular project. This evidence aims to provide a grant committee that your project can be accomplished based on previous studies that were successful. This will bolster the reputation of your research group and your area of study and make it more likely for your project to be funded. If the study has preliminary data which is promising, it may also be discussed here.

Other factors that should be mentioned include participants in the investigating team, ethics approval status, details on the test subjects, previous funding, significance of data for outcomes, and the timeframe for results and updates. Each section should be organized into individual sub-headings. The formatting for this will be contingent on the particular grant application as they may be different for each application.

It should be noted that if your project involves working with living human or animal participants, there should be a segment that discusses how your project will manage their care/treatment throughout the research project. While the project itself may have ethical approval, the individual grant may have their own moral ideas on how their care or investigations should be managed. It may be worth mentioning how the participants would be treated in an ethical manner. This is especially important in community proposals.

19.10 Concluding Part

The conclusion for any grant proposal is self-explanatory and should be short, simple, and to the point. This is a two to three paragraph to summaries the importance of the project and why it needs to be funded. Not every proposal will require a conclusion, but it serves as a useful reminder to the reader as to what the project aims to accomplish.

19.11 Conclusion

Australian government bodies, private companies, and charities are good sources of grants to fund any research projects. Applications for individual grants are variable in their required content and formatting. While this chapter provides a general overview as to what would be required, it is still crucial to conduct one's own research into their own project requirements and also the individual grant requirements. A successful application will generate the project funding within that grant period, usually the following year, so it is important to plan ahead. A piece of general advice is to apply broadly and check up on the applications frequently in order to avoid being under-funded or missing important deadlines.

Case Scenario
A researcher is investigating the utility of a newly discovered urinary test as a screening tool for prostate cancer. The project will require a lot of funding to conduct the tests, report on the data and follow-up the patients. In order to get funding from the NHMRC, a grant proposal must be submitted. Given this is a clinical trial, the funding will come from the "Clinical Trial and Cohort Studies Grant." The supporting components commonly expected are:

- Principle supervisor details including license for your study.
- Grant proposal including a brief explanation of your project and what it aims to achieve.
- Overview of the budget for the study and expected expenses.
- Current funding sources.
- Any conflicts of interest.

Consider the main parts of a grant proposal for a clinical trial like this
- The introduction including the impact of the disease in society and the importance of early screening.
- The current evidence for your study.
- The requirement for funding including what the expected expenditure on this study will be.
- The long-term benefits (both societal and monetary) to funding a trial like this.

References

1. Australian Bureau of Statistics. Research and Experimental Development, Government and Private Non-Profit Organisations, Australia [Updated 2019]. https://www.abs.gov.au/statistics/industry/technology-and-innovation/research-and-experimental-development-government-and-private-non-profit-organisations-australia/latest-release.
2. Sohn E. Secrets to writing a winning grant. Nature. 2020;577(7788):133–5.
3. National Health and Medical Research Council. Development Grants for funding commencing in 2021, Australian Government. Canberra: National Health and Medical Research Council; 2020.
4. Planning and Writing a Grant Proposal [Internet]. University of Wisconsin: Madison [Updated 7/12/2017]. https://writing.wisc.edu/handbook/assignments/grants-2/#6.
5. Australian Institute of Aboriginal and Torres Strait Islander Studies [Internet]. Current Projects [Updated 2021]. https://aiatsis.gov.au/research/current-projects.
6. Pzifer's Competitive Grants Program [Internet]. Pzifer. [Updated 2021]. https://www.pfizer.com/purpose/independent-grants/competitive-grants.
7. Grant Proposals (or Give Me the Money!) [Internet]. University of North Carolina at Chapel Hill. [Updated 2021]. https://writingcenter.unc.edu/tips-and-tools/grant-proposals-or-give-me-the-money/.
8. Grants-in-Aids [Internet]. Cancer Council Victoria. [Updated 2021]. https://www.cancervic.org.au/research/grants/grants-in-aid.

Proposal Writing for Grant Application in Malaysia

20

Wei Hong Lai, Alan Yean Yip Fong, and Asri bin Said

> *Never hesitate to go far away, beyond all seas, all frontiers, all countries, all beliefs*
>
> *Amin Maalouf*

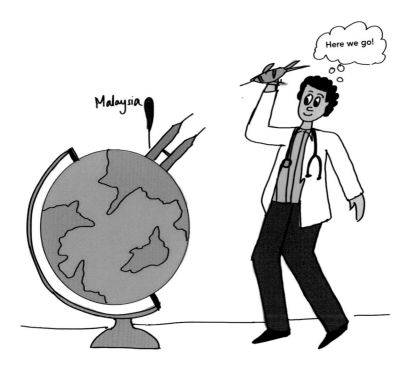

Proposal writing for grant application in Malaysia

W. H. Lai (✉)
Clinical Research Centre, Institute for Clinical Research, Sarawak General Hospital, Jalan Hospital, Kuching, Sarawak, Malaysia

Objectives

- To provide a guideline to the reader on drafting a winning research proposal for grant application in Malaysia.
- To provide an overview of available research grants in Malaysia [Ministry of Science, Technology, and Innovation (MOSTI), Ministry of Health (MOH), and Ministry of Higher Education (MOHE)].
- To provide technical advice on how to prepare a proposal with or without commercial outcomes and identify suitable grants.

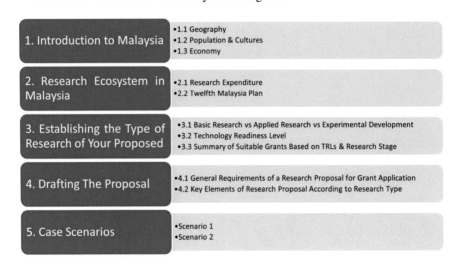

Flow chart depicting the important content of the chapter

20.1 Introduction to Malaysia

20.1.1 Geography

Malaysia is located within Southeast Asia, and its western border is with Thailand in the north and Singapore in the south, while its eastern border is with Brunei and Indonesia. Malaysia represents the best of Asia because being strategically positioned in the heart of Southeast Asia.

A. Y. Y. Fong
Clinical Research Centre, Institute for Clinical Research, Sarawak General Hospital, Jalan Hospital, Kuching, Sarawak, Malaysia

Sarawak Heart Centre, Kuching-Samarahan Expressway, Kota Samarahan, Sarawak, Malaysia

A. b. Said
Sarawak Heart Centre, Kuching-Samarahan Expressway, Kota Samarahan, Sarawak, Malaysia

Faculty of Medicine and Health Sciences, University Malaysia Sarawak, Jalan Datuk Mohammad Musa, Kota Samarahan, Sarawak, Malaysia

20.1.2 Population and Cultures

Malaysia is a multiethnic and multicultural federation of 13 states and 3 federal territories. The Department of Statistic Malaysia released the estimates of population in 2020 to be approximately 32.6 million, which consisted of 25.4 million of this population residing in urban areas. This means that most Malaysian were residing in urban areas throughout the 13 states. Of a total of 29.7 million Malaysian citizens, a large percentage (69.6%) of it comprised the Bumiputera, with the major group of these Bumiputera being ethnic Malays, trailed by non-Malay indigenous groups from north Borneo (i.e., Sabah) and Sarawak, as well as the Orang Asli. Then, the Chinese comprised 22.6% of these citizens, along with Indians being 6.8% and other ethnic minorities being 1.0% of these citizens. As for their religious faiths, there was approximately 61.3% of the Malaysian population practiced Islam, along with 19.8% practicing Buddhism, 9.2% practicing Christianity, 6.3% practicing Hinduism, 1.3% practicing other traditional Chinese religions, and 0.7% reported having no religion. A final remaining 1.4% of the population does not state their religious conviction [1].

20.1.3 Economy

Malaysia has the infrastructure, connectivity, and an increasingly agile and adaptable talent pool because of its strategic location in the center of the Association of Southeast Asian Nations (ASEAN) [2]. According to the recent World Bank Report, Malaysia is one of the world's most competitive economies; and since 2010, with Gross Domestic Product (GDP) ratio has averaged above 130% [3]. Competitive market with strong promotion of foreign investment is instrumental in creating employment opportunities that spur income growth, with at least 40% of local jobs in Malaysia involved with export businesses, offering employment possibilities that stimulate income development [3]. Malaysia's economy has been on an upward trend since the Asian financial crisis (1997–1998), with an average growth of 5.4% since 2010; as a result, Malaysia's shift from an upper-middle-income to a high-income economy is scheduled to be achieved by 2024 [3].

20.2 Research Ecosystem in Malaysia

20.2.1 Research Expenditure

20.2.1.1 International Comparison of Research and Development (R & D) Expenditure

According to a published Malaysian report, the USA rated first among nations in the Organization for Economic Co-operation and Development (OECD) with USD 543,249 million being spent on R & D activities, followed by Japan with USD 170,901 million and Germany with USD 131,339 million. The top five OECD countries with the highest R & D expenditure were the USA, Japan, Germany, South Korea, and France while Malaysia ranked 18th in R & D expenditure [4].

20.2.1.2 Overview of R & D Activities in Malaysia

The National Survey of R & D 2019 findings had reported that an increasing trend of Basic Research and Experimental Development continued persistently and Applied Research had shown a decreasing trend. It should be noted that Basic Research was mostly contributed by Higher Learning institutions (HLI) and Applied Research and Experimental Development were mainly contributed by Business Enterprises (BE). In 2018, both Basic Research and Applied Research were receiving an almost equal share of R & D funding; with Medical and Health Sciences activities contributing 8.9% in the total Field of Research (FOR) [4].

20.2.1.3 Gross Expenditure on Research and Development (GERD)

Malaysia's overall gross domestic expenditure on research and development (GERD) is expected to be RM 15,060 million in 2018, which had shown a decline of approximately RM 2,625 million as compared with RM 17,685 in 2016. Approximately 82% of GERD is being spent on current expenditure and 18% of GERD is being spent on capital [4].

20.2.2 Twelfth Malaysia Plan (12MP)

The Malaysia Plan (also known as the Malaysia 5-Year Plan) is a detailed summary of the government's development plans and initiatives. The first Malaysia Plan was established in 1965, and it covered the whole government's development plan from 1966 to 1970. Currently, Malaysia is having its Twelfth Malaysia Plan (12MP) which is designed to align Malaysia with the shared prosperity initiative that encompasses three aspects, namely: social re-engineering, environmental sustainability, and economic empowerment [5]. In this chapter, guidelines for grant proposal writing will be discussed according to selected 12MP grants from the Ministry of Science, Technology, and Innovation (MOSTI), Ministry of Health (MOH), and Ministry of Higher Education (MOHE).

20.2.2.1 MOSTI's Malaysia Grand Challenge (MGC)

MOSTI launched the Malaysia Grand Challenge (MGC) on 8 January 2021, with the aim to elevate the National Science, Technology, and Innovation agenda to enhance a sustainable and inclusive economy in line with the Science, Technology, and Innovation Policy (DSTIN) for 2021 to 2030. MGC seeks to promote the Malaysian researchers in pursuing quality and high-impact research according to the priority areas that have been identified through the 10–10 Malaysian Science, Technology, Innovation and Economy (MySTIE) framework as well as the 30 Niche Areas that have been identified. There are 5 grants for this initiative and they are: (1) Applied Innovation Fund, (2) Technology Development Fund 1, (3) Technology Development Fund 2, (4) Bridging Fund, and (5) MOSTI Combating COVID-19.

10–10 Malaysian Science, Technology, Innovation, and Economy (MySTIE) Framework

10–10 MySTIE Framework was established by the Academy of Sciences Malaysia with the aim to catalyst socioeconomic transformation by introducing a total of 30 National STIE Areas of Specialization with 6 core components, along with its 20 strategies and 46 initiatives that covered all essential sectors and involving people from all walks of life [6]. The 10 priority areas are energy, biodiversity and environment, education, tourism and arts, forestry and agriculture, food and water, medicine and health care, culture, transportation and smart cities, business and financial services, and smart systems and technologies. These priority areas will complement the 10 science and technology drivers such as blockchain, 5G/6G, advanced intelligence systems, and others. Hence, the purpose of launching the MySTIE 10–10 is to integrate 10 global science and technology drivers with 10 socioeconomic drivers in the country so that science, technology, innovation (STI), and social sciences can complement each other. By integrating the two major sectors of STI and economics; it is then possible to utilize STI as a tool to address national issues and challenges, and then to move Malaysia up in the global value chain in technological innovation.

20.2.2.2 MOHE's Malaysia Greater Research Network System (MyGRANTS)

Malaysia Greater Research Network System (MyGRANTS) is a web-based system designed and developed by MOHE to assist researchers in research-related matters and activities [7]. One of its main functions is to provide a platform to all researchers (particularly those under the purview of MOHE) for the application of various MOHE research grants; and grants available for application at the time of writing are (1) Fundamental Research Grant Scheme (FRGS), (2) Prototype Development Research Grant Scheme (PRGS), (3) Trans-Disciplinary Research Grant Scheme (TRGS), (4) Long-Term Research Grant Scheme (LRGS), (5) *Geran Sanjungan Penyelidikan KPM* (*GSP-KPM*), (6) Research Acculturation Collaborative Effort (RACE), and (7) Malaysia Laboratories for Academia-Business Collaboration (MyLAB) [7].

20.2.2.3 MOH's Research Grant (MRG)

MOH Research Grant (MRG) supports medical and health sciences research initiatives that are aligned with national priorities, with objectives to (1) develop new scientific information in order to enhance health and healthcare delivery and (2) to support and finance R & D initiatives that will result in new information and discoveries that will help to spur the development of innovative technologies and processes [8].

20.3 Establishing the Type of Research (and Technology Readiness Level, If Applicable) of Your Proposed Research Idea

20.3.1 Basic Research vs Applied Research vs Experimental Development

R & D activities could be categorized to Basic Research, Applied Research, and Experimental Development and their definition according to Frascati Manual (2015) are listed in Table 20.1 [4].

It is essential for a researcher to understand the differences in the listed research type and to have a clear idea what is the research goal(s) that the researcher is set to achieve, in order to determine suitable funding source and their scopes of funding.

20.3.2 Technology Readiness Level (TRL)

The utilization of technology readiness levels (TRLs) began with the National Aeronautics and Space Administration (NASA) in the 1970s as an approach to monitoring and determining the maturity of aerospace technology and its associated device(s) [9]. Over the years, the use of NASA's 9-tier scale has expanded to other industries to monitor the status of emerging technologies [10]. The degree to which technology has matured and its commercial readiness will be evaluated, and a TRL grade was issued based on the following:

TRL 1: Basic/fundamental principle(s)/concept(s) observed and reported.

TRL 2: Technology principle(s)/concept(s) and/or application(s) formulated.

TRL 3: Analytical and experimental critical function(s) and/or characteristic proof-of-concept(s).

TRL 4: Component(s) and/or breadboard(s) validation in laboratory environment/setting.

TRL 5: Component(s) and/or breadboard(s) validation in relevant environment/setting.

Table 20.1 Type of research

Basic research	Applied research	Experimental development
"Experimental or theoretical work undertaken primarily to acquire new knowledge of the underlying foundation of phenomena and observable facts, without any particular application or use in view"	"Original investigation was undertaken in order to acquire new knowledge. It is, however, directed primarily towards a specific, practical aim or objective"	"Systematic work, drawing on knowledge gained from research and practical experience and producing additional knowledge, which is directed to producing new products or processes or to improving existing products or processes"

TRL 6: System/subsystem model(s) or prototype(s) demonstration in a relevant environment/setting (ground or space).

TRL 7: System prototype(s) demonstration in a space environment/setting.

TRL 8: Actual system concluded and "flight qualified" by means of trial and error (ground or space).

TRL 9: Actual system "flight proven" via successful mission operators.

20.3.2.1 Utilization of TRL in Malaysia

In Malaysia, NASA's TRL has been adapted into its R, D, and C & I landscape. MOSTI has defined the TRLs for Malaysia Commercialization Year as follows [11]:

TRL 1: Promising research funding.

TRL 2: Technology application formulated.

TRL 3: Lab-scale experimental proof of concept.

TRL 4: Lab-scale development and integration.

TRL 5: Production enhancement/techno-economic model.

TRL 6: Scale-up and pilot-scale technology validation.

TRL 7: Detailed engineering/plant design.

TRL 8: Semi-works scale technology demonstration.

TRL 9: Large-scale commercial operations.

In addition, all the TRLs were grouped into three stages:

Discovery Stage

TRL 1–3: Basic research
   TRL 4: Feasibility demonstration
   TRL 5: Technology development
   TRL 6: Viability demonstration

Determination Stage

TRL 7–8: Commercial transition

Development Stage

TRL 9: Commercial deployment

Therefore, researchers applying for Malaysia grant with technology must first establish the TRL of their research and determine the suitable grant based on their proposed research idea.

20.3.3 Summary of Suitable Grants Based on TRLs and Research Stage

In this section, selected grants from MOSTI, MOHE, and MOH will be summarized in Table 20.2 together with their TRL, if applicable. Most of the listed MOHE grants and MOH grants are suitable for Discovery Stage while most of the listed MOSTI funds are suitable for pre-commercialization activities. Pre-commercialization

Table 20.2 Summary of selected grants and mapping of their TRL

Ministry	Grant	Aim of grant	Scope of funding and criteria	TRL
MOHE	Fundamental Research Grant Scheme (FRGS)	This grant aims to accelerate the generation of theories, concepts, and new ideas as a catalyst for new discoveries which breaks through the boundaries of knowledge and innovative creation	Refer to their official application guidelines available at this link: http://mygrants.gov.my	Not described in guidelines (based on writers' comprehension, suitable for discovery stage)
	Prototype Development Research Grant Scheme (PRGS)	This grant aims to help bridge the gap between research findings and commercialization for the purpose of the creation of new technologies/discoveries molded-in Malaysia in accordance with the K-Economy's requirements and the New Economic Model's implementation	Refer to their official application guidelines available at this link: http://mygrants.gov.my	3–5
	Trans-Disciplinary Research Grant Scheme (TRGS)	This grant aspires to speed the development of new theories, concepts, and ideas that may serve as a springboard for new discoveries that push the frontiers of knowledge and inventive innovation	Refer to their official application guidelines available at this link: http://mygrants.gov.my	Not described in guidelines (based on writers' comprehension, suitable for TRL 1–8)
	Long-Term Research Grant Scheme (LRGS)	This grant aims to strengthen excellence in the generation of theories, new ideas, and innovative creations that are at the forefront in strategic fields for the development of knowledge frontiers	Refer to their official application guidelines available at this link: http://mygrants.gov.my	Not described in guidelines (based on writers' comprehension, suitable for discovery stage)

	Malaysia Laboratories for Academia-Business Collaboration (MyLAB)	The MyLAB program aims to develop and consolidate research-based products with high potential for commercialization in strategic thrust areas	Refer to their official application guidelines available at this link: http://mygrants.gov.my	6–7
MOH	MOH Research Grant	This grant aims to (1) generate new scientific knowledge to improve health and improve health delivery services; and (2) support and fund R & D projects to generate new knowledge and discoveries that can catalyze the development of innovative technologies and processes	Refer to their official application guidelines available at this link: https://www.nmrr.gov.my/doc/ Garis-Panduan-Institut-Kesihatan-Negara-NIH-Mengenai-Permohonan-Geran-Penyelidikan-KKM.pdf	Not described in guidelines (based on writers' comprehension, suitable for discovery stage)
MOSTI	Applied Innovation Fund	This grant aims to increase the participation of innovators in innovative activities and encourage the development of new goods, processes, systems, or services that have the potential to be commercialized via technical innovation	Refer to their official application guidelines available at this link: https://edana.mosti.gov.my/	2–4
	Technology Development Fund 1	This grant aims to: (1) develop existing concepts related to the design of technologies, processes, or products that have the potential to be commercialized; and (2) promote the expansion of research and technology development among Government Research Institutes, STI Agencies, Higher Education Institutions and Industry	Refer to their official application guidelines available at this link: https://edana.mosti.gov.my/	2–4

(continued)

Table 20.2 (continued)

Ministry	Grant	Aim of grant	Scope of funding and criteria	TRL
	Technology Development Fund 2	This grant aims to: (1) develop existing concepts related to the design of technologies, processes, or products towards commercialization to reduce the gap of failure (valley of death) and (2) promote the expansion of research and technology development by establishing a network of collaboration between Government Research Institutes, Government STI agencies, higher education institutions and industry	Refer to their official application guidelines available at this link: https://edana.mosti.gov.my/	4–7
	Bridging Fund	This grant aims to: (1) reduce the failure gap (valley of death) between pre-commercialization and commercialization and (2) improve R & D product readiness in order to access the market	Refer to their official application guidelines available at this link: https://edana.mosti.gov.my/	7–9
	MOSTI Combating Covid-19	This grant aims to combat the spread of the COVID-19 pandemic	Refer to their official application guidelines available at this link: https://edana.mosti.gov.my/	2–9

(Information on listed grants is correct and has been verified at the time of writing)

activities are actions that are undertaken before the real active commercialization phase and are aimed towards the effective commercialization of a technology or knowledge asset, either internally or externally [12].

20.4 Drafting the Proposal

20.4.1 General Requirements of a Research Proposal for Grant Application

According to Monavarian (2021), a grant proposal is a formal document that you draft to achieve a specific aim(s) and to be submitted to the relevant funding agency or an investing organization to convince them to provide the requested financial support by showing that (1) you have a viable plan for pursuing a particular research goal and (2) that the team is fully capable of accomplishing the proposed goals [13]. In addition, it is essential to include a description of the proposed research ideas and preliminary results (if applicable) relative to the proposed goals and budget plans [13]. Therefore, in order to begin with a description of a successful grant application, it is necessary to revisit the fundamental elements in drafting a grant proposal, to ensure a feasible and scientifically valid research grant proposal will be drafted. Information on the fundamental of a grant proposal can be referred to in Chapter "What is a grant? How to prepare for writing a grant proposal application."

20.4.2 Key Elements of Research Proposal According to Research Type

20.4.2.1 Research Focused on Knowledge Generation and Policy-Driven

This category usually involves both basic and applied research. It is essential for a researcher to be able to determine whether the proposed research is basic and applied research so that he/she is able to incorporate the required weightage and rationale of the anticipated research proposal according to its type of research. As described in Table 20.1, basic research is a research with the aim to generate new knowledge and/or expand the existing knowledge-base of a certain field without regard to any specific application or usage; and usually involves the exploration and/or explanation of a specific topic in-depth with the ambition to generate new knowledge (and/or expand existing knowledge) to decrease existing knowledge gap. In medical and health sciences, basic research plays a significant role in the understanding and interpretation of medical and healthcare issues. Basic research allows medical and scientific communities to gain more insight into the origin and pathogenesis of the disease(s), and generated knowledge from basic research has been attributed to several medical breakthroughs which contributed to rapid progress in global health. Examples of basic research in medical and health sciences include:

1. Investigation to determine the symptoms caused by Nipah virus (*Nipah henipavirus*) infection.
2. Investigation to identify genetic variant(s) involved in the pathogenesis of Nasopharyngeal Carcinoma (NPC).

Additionally, as described in Table 20.1, applied research is a form of an investigation conducted to generate new knowledge with the aim to provide a solution(s) to raised inquiry and/or a particular problem. On many occasions, this form of investigation normally employs empirical methodologies and may act as the continuance research design pursuant to basic research as it generates solution(s) to a specific inquiry and/or a particular problem by incorporating findings concluded from basic research [14]. In medical and health sciences, this form of investigation can be referred to as applied clinical research and is normally employed to determine the degree to which the findings of concluded basic research could be utilized. Examples of applied research in medical and health sciences include:

1. Investigation to identify the optimal approach to manage patients with drug-induced lung diseases with pre-existing renal impairment.
2. Investigation to identify the optimal approach to treat patients with iatrogenic and drug-induced hypertension.

Hence, the key focus for a researcher when drafting basic or applied research should be on its theoretical framework and the development of a theoretical framework involves the determination of the research question and its fundamental theory, identification of key variables, and the relationships among them, and the evaluation of hypothesis [15].

20.4.2.2 Research with a Commercial Outcome

Medical and health researchers are increasingly encouraged to focus on devising a plan for the commercialization of their research findings and/or research output. Pre-commercialization is to establish a link between basic/applied research with technology commercialization [16]. When drafting a grant proposal for research that focuses on commercialization, the major considerations are:

1. Technology: This includes the uniqueness and/or innovativeness and/or inventiveness of the proposed developed technology to ensure the submitted proposal is original and able to pioneer a niche segment, and this section could be supported with a patent search result. In addition, it is essential to ensure the project objectives are viable and the methodology is suitable to exert strong confidence in the completion of proposed activities. Furthermore, to convince the reviewer of the potential of the proposed idea to be able to be scaled, it is paramount to also include information on the manufacturability together with regulatory compliance and applicable standard.

2. Commercial potential: In order to portray the commercial potential for proposed technology, it is necessary to include information such as the market potential and demand for proposed technology and its appropriateness of time to market, sustainability of proposed technology, and its cost-effectiveness, diffusion, marketing strategy with the business model and its potential diffusion into the different market segment.
3. Financial and management: This includes information on the potential to generate a return on investment (ROI) and the value for money for the proposed technology, including social return on investment (SROI). Additionally, it is essential to describe the significance and relevance of key milestones, together with its risk management plan.

20.5   Case Scenarios

Due to the differing requirements imposed by the category of research, a major consideration for the preparation of a research proposal to be submitted for a grant application is the establishment of the type of research (and TRL, if applicable) as described in Sect. 20.3 (in this chapter) and determine the suitable grant based on proposed research idea. Furthermore, the proposal should be prepared and submitted according to the requirements of the funding provider (Table 20.2). Additionally, it must be emphasized that under all circumstances, the appropriate choice of a specific type of research grant for a grant application to apply for shall ultimately depend on the eligibility criteria imposed by each type of research grant, i.e., only MOH staff are eligible to apply for MRG.

In this section, simple reference steps (Fig. 20.1) are introduced as a guide for grant applicants and the following are two examples of how a grant application can determine which type of research grant is more suitable and draft a proposal based on key elements.

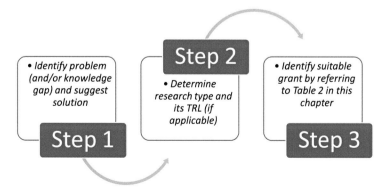

Fig. 20.1 Steps to determine a suitable grant for the proposed research

Scenario 1

Step 1: Identify the problem (and/or knowledge gap) and suggest a solution

Problem/knowledge gap: Prevalence of Nasopharyngeal Carcinoma (NPC) incidence is higher in Bidayuh and Iban tribes in Sarawak, health and scientific communities are unsure if this was contributed (fully or partly) by specific genetic variant(s).

Proposed solution: Therefore, to obtain an answer to the above question, the grant applicant decided to conduct a targeted genomic sequencing to identify genetic variant(s) involved in the pathogenesis of NPC and determine whether identified genetic variant(s) is/are a tribe (and ethnic) specific.

Step 2: Determine the research type and its TRL (if applicable)

The objective of the proposed research is to generate genomic evidence on whether genetic variant(s) specific to Bidayuh and Iban tribes in Sarawak involve in the pathogenesis of NPC. Therefore, this is basic research and generated genomic evidence will contribute to new knowledge.

Step 3: Identify a suitable grant by referring to Table 20.2

This is basic research, and it seems FRGS and MRG are most suitable. Hence, the proposal should be drafted in accordance with FRGS or MRG requirements. In addition to the basic elements outlined in Chapter "Checklist for grant proposal—Mandatory elements," the grant applicant will need to emphasize the theoretical framework of the proposed research, as discussed in Sect. 20.4.2.1 Research focused on knowledge generation and policy driven in this chapter.

Scenario 2

Step 1: Identify the problem (and/or knowledge gap) and suggest a solution

Problem/knowledge gap: Antiviral drugs for human immunodeficiency virus (HIV) are now losing their effectiveness because HIV has now begun to develop resistance to them.

Proposed solution: Therefore, to provide alternative antiviral drug(s) for HIV treatment, the grant applicant decided to conduct research with the aim to discover new bioactive compound(s) from the plant(s) potential to be developed as an alternative antiviral drug(s) for HIV treatment.

Step 2: Determine the research type and its TRL (if applicable)

At present, bioactive compound(s) from the plant(s) which show potential for development into a new antiviral drug(s) for HIV treatment have been identified. Proof-of-concept (PoC) has been successfully conducted and present findings require lab-scale development and integration. Hence, the proposed research has completed/reached TRL 3, and moving towards TRL 4.

Step 3: Identify a suitable grant by referring to Table 20.2

This research is intended to develop a novel product and then mass produces and disseminates it as an alternative antiviral drug(s) for HIV treatment. At present, the proposed research activities are at the pre-commercialization stage (i.e., TRL 4) and are more suited to MOHE's PRGS and MOSTI's Applied Innovative Fund, Technology Development Fund 1, and Technology Development Fund 2. Hence, the proposal should be drafted in accordance with the requirements of the selected grant.

In addition to the basic elements outlined in Chapter "Checklist for grant proposal—Mandatory elements,", the grant applicant will need to emphasize the technology and commercial viability of the proposed research, as discussed in Sect. 20.4.2.2 Research with commercial outcome in this chapter.

20.6 Responsibilities of Grant Recipient

Overall, a grant recipient has a responsibility to ensure that the grant funding must be spent on only the listed activities which are permitted by the funding agency and also that must be solely for the purpose of completion of the research work outlined by a grant proposal. In addition, every recipient of a research grant will be required to strictly comply with the laws of the country, the income tax department of the country, and any other relevant authorities relating to the use of the funds.

20.7 Conclusion

It is paramount to identify suitable grant and communicate your research ideas efficiently to grant provider. Hence, most of the suggestions in this guide are intended to enhance the clarity with which your application is presented to grant provider. Additionally, a well-written application also emphasizes order and attention to detail.

References

1. Amin L, Olesen A, Mahadi Z, Ibrahim M. Current status and future challenges of biobank research in Malaysia. Asian Bioeth Rev. 2021;13:297–315. https://doi.org/10.1007/s41649-021-00171-5.
2. MDEC. Introduction to Malaysia. 2021. https://mdec.my/about-malaysia/introduction/. Accessed 23 Jul 2021.
3. World Bank Group. Malaysia Economic Monitor: Weathering the Surge [Internet]. 2021. https://openknowledge.worldbank.org/handle/10986/35812.
4. MOSTI. National Survey of Research and Development (R & D) in Malaysia 2019 [Internet]. 2020. https://mastic.mosti.gov.my/sti-survey-content-spds/national-survey-research-and-development-rd-2019.
5. EPU. Twelfth Malaysia Plan, 2021–2025 [Internet]. 2021. https://rmke12.epu.gov.my/. Accessed 23 Jul 2021.
6. Academy of Sciences Malaysia. 10 Malaysian Science, Technology, Innovation and Economy (MySTIE) Framework. 2020.
7. MOE. Malaysia Greater Research Network System (MyGRANTS) [Internet]. 2021. https://www.mohe.gov.my/en/services/research/mygrants. Accessed 23 Jul 2021.
8. MOSTI. MOH Research Grant (MRG) [Internet]. 2021. https://mastic.mosti.gov.my/sti-incentive/moh-research-grant-mrg. Accessed 23 Jul 2021.
9. TWI. What are Technology Readiness Levels (TRL)? [Internet]. 2021. https://www.twi-global.com/technical-knowledge/faqs/technology-readiness-levels. Accessed 23 Jul 2021.

10. TEMPO. Understanding Technology Readiness Level for Medical Devices Development [Internet]. 2021. https://www.tempoautomation.com/blog/understanding-technology-readiness-level-for-medical-devices-development/. Accessed 23 Jul 2021.
11. MOSTI. Technology Readiness Levels [Internet]. 2021. https://mcyportal.mosti.gov.my/web/tips-panduan/technology-readiness-level-trl/. Accessed 23 Jul 2021.
12. Kutvonen A, Torkkeli MT, Lin B. Pre-commercialisation activities in external exploitation of technology. Int J Innov Learn. 2010;8(2):208–30.
13. Monavarian M. Basics of scientific and technical writing: grant proposals. MRS Bull. 2021;46: 1–3. https://doi.org/10.1557/s43577-021-00105-4.
14. Baimyrzaeva M. Beginners' guide for applied research process: what is it, and why and how to do it? Univ Cent Asia Grad Sch Dev. 2018;4:1–43.
15. Pequegnat W, Stover E, Boyce CA. How to write a successful research grant application. 2nd ed. Cham: Springer; 2011. p. 283.
16. Keswani C, Sarma BK, Singh HB. Agriculturally important microorganisms as biofertilizers: commercialization and regulatory requirements in Asia. In: Agriculturally important microorganisms. Singapore: Springer; 2016. p. 1–305.

Grant Writing for Other Asian Countries

21

Devyani Sharma, Upninder Kaur, Rakesh Sehgal,
and Subhash Chandra Parija

> *Climb the mountain, not so the world can see you, but so you can see the world*
>
> *David McCullough Jr.*

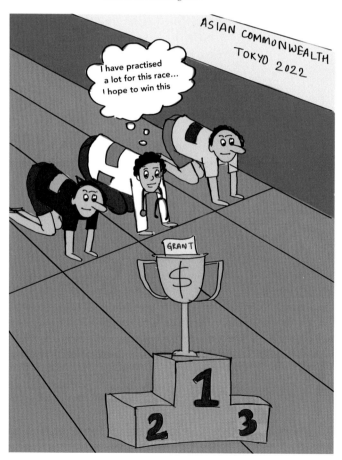

Grant writing for other Asian countries

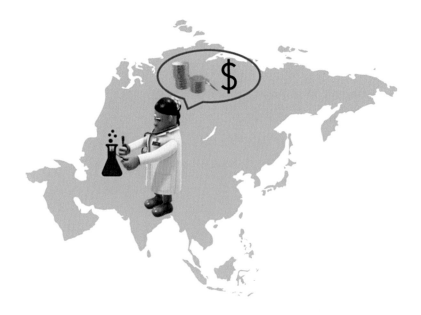

Objectives
- Understand the role of funding in promulgating research in Asian countries
- Be aware of the various international and region-specific bodies offering grants

21.1   Introduction

Medical education and related health sciences research contribute significantly to the country's economic development, resulting in long-term sustainable growth and eventually an improvement in health care and living standards [1]. With 4.40 billion inhabitants, Asia is the world's largest and most populous continent. Northern Asia, Western Asia, Central Asia, Eastern Asia, Southern Asia and Southeast Asia are the subregions, respectively. Among these China, Georgia, Israel, Japan and India are the top five nations in Asia for medical education and research wheras Yemen, Palestine, Myanmar, Kazakhstan, Syria and Armenia are among the countries with the lowest rankings in research [2]. Stewardship, financing, human and institutional capability, improvement and implementation of research are the four core components of health research systems. Out of all these financing has a crucial

D. Sharma · U. Kaur · R. Sehgal (✉)
Department of Medical Parasitology, Postgraduate Institute of Medical Education and Research (PGIMER), Chandigarh, India

S. C. Parija
Sri Balaji Vidyapeeth, Pondicherry, India

role to play. Despite Asia's large disease burden, research is sometimes seen as an expense rather than an investment, resulting in research programs that are mostly funded by outside sources. In many countries, such as Nepal and Bangladesh, a lack of funding is the fundamental barrier to health research, therefore financial and technical aid from outside sources is regarded as valuable [3]. Considering this grant writing is critical and has an important role to play.

21.2   Where and How to being With?

As Vincent van Gogh has quoted, "The beginning is perhaps more difficult than anything else, but keep heart, it will turn out all right." as. As a matter of fact, the first step is to become familiar with the many sorts of grants that are available in a certain area. Both national and regional funding sources fall under this category. The one that would support your study plan must then be chosen after sorting them according to your specified preferences. The majority of funding organisations present the main idea of the research proposal grant that they seek to sponsor when their portals open at predetermined times. For instance, at appropriate dates, the Indian Council for Medical Research, New Delhi, India, announces call for proposals that emphasises the core concept of the proposal they intend to fund. The research calls specifically cover drug development, parasite epidemiology, medical diagnostics and many other facets of medical research. Understanding and keeping a record of the various openings of the funding organisations can help you create a basic structure for a research proposal grant that can then be modified in response to the call made. Grants are granted to individuals conducting research, Ph.D. students and others who desire to enter and carry out research in general.

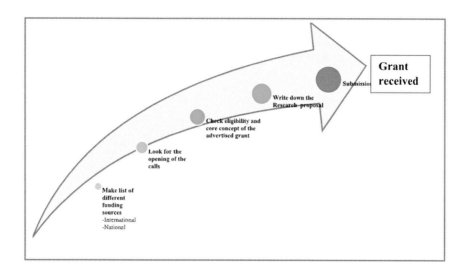

21.3   Grant Categories

There are four types of grants available—competitive funding, formula funding, continuation funding and pass-through funding [4].

- **Competitive funding**: After the possible recipients have submitted their ideas, the reviewers make a decision based on the proposal.
- **Formula funding**: It is predetermined that the beneficiary will receive the funds as long as the grant criteria are met.
- **Continuation funding**: It is given for multi-year research and is renewed on an annual basis.
- **Pass-through funding**: An intermediary is used to deliver the grant from an organization to the beneficiary.

For Asian countries, medical research grants are available both from international and Specific Regional Institutes/Departments. As the Asian subcontinent is primarily made up of developing countries, several funds from international sources are awarded to well-written research applications that address critical health issues affecting the country's growth.

21.4   Major International Funding Sources

Funds can be obtained from a variety of international sources. The award amount is substantial and the possibilities are limitless. Through their grant procedures, the National Institute on Deafness and Other Communication Disorders funds a wide range of research. This covers research grants, research training, career development awards, small company grants, clinical research center grants, conference grants, administrative supplements and drug development financing [5]. Other financial grants, such as those from the European Commission, the World Health Organization and others, are similar. The following are a few of the prominent international funding organizations [6, 7].

- Pasteur Institute
- SIDA—The Swedish International Development Cooperation Agency
- SRC—Semiconductor Research Centre
- USAID—United States Agency for International Development
- The Wellcome Trust
- EDCTP—European and Developing Countries Clinical Trials
- GACD—Global Alliance for Chronic Diseases
- MRC—Medical Research Council
- NIH—National Institute of Health
- WHO—World Health Organization
- AMED—The Japan Agency for Medical Research and Development
- BMBF—Federal Ministry of Education and Research
- CIHR—Canadian Institute of Health Research

- EC—European Commission
- HHMI—Howard Hughes Medical Institute
- DFID—Department for International Development
- Ford Foundation
- Rockefeller Foundation
- The Fleming fund

21.5 Regional Grants Sources

These are the financing institutes or organizations that finance grant submissions from a specific region, such as the Southeast Asia One Health University Network, which funds research in Southeast Asian countries. Below are listed a few of the funding sources in different regions of Asia. Writing a grant proposal for a regional funding source follows a similar principle and approach; however, there are a few key factors to remember (Table 21.1).

21.6 Description of a Few Regional Grants Funding Sources

1. SEAOHUN—This refers to the Southeast Asia One Health University network. Their small grants program primarily funds submissions that are focused on a single health approach. You must be a SEAOHUN faculty member or a health professional from one of the member nations to be eligible in order to apply for a research grant [8].
2. Russian Foundation for Basic Research—It is a funding body of the Russian government. It provides funding to both individual scientists as well as research teams [9].
3. National Natural Science Foundation of China—It is managed by China's Ministry of Science and Technology. Their primary goal is to provide funding for basic and applied research in China [9].
4. Global Health Research Centre of Central Asia—. The centres headquarters are based in Kazakhstan. The scope of research proposals here is broad encompassing HIV/AIDS, malnutrition and many other issues, particularly those which are predominant in Central Asian countries. The National Institute of Health, as well as a few local sources, are also funding the research [10].
5. Japan Agency for Medical Research and Development—It focuses on medical research, which ranges from basic research to clinical trials [11].
6. Qatar National Research Fund—It is situated in Qatar and intends to sponsor selected research in a variety of sectors including health sciences, biological sciences, social sciences and others [12].
7. Bangladesh Medical Research Council—It is a national research organization in Bangladesh that funds medical research. It has recently taken the initiative to launch the Bangladesh Cancer Genome Project, which will profile cancer in the region [13].

Table 21.1 Regional grants sources

Northern Asia (Russia, Mongolia, Japan, Korea and China)	• China Medical Board • National Natural Science Foundation of China • Russian Academy of Sciences • Russian Foundation for Basic Research • Japan Agency for Medical Research and Development • Japan Science and Technology Agency • National Research Foundation Korea
Central Asia (Kazakhstan, Kyrgyz Republic, Tajikistan, Turkmenistan and Uzbekistan)	• Nazarbayev University • Central Asia Medical Education Initiative • Global Health Research Centre of Central Asia
Eastern Asia (China, Hong Kong, Japan, Macau, Mongolia, North Korea, South Korea and Taiwan)	• Japan Agency for Medical Research and Development • Japan Science and Technology Agency • Health and Medical Research Fund, Hong Kong • National Research Foundation of Korea • National Health Research Institutes, Taiwan • Seoul National University Asia Centre
Western Asia (Bahrain, Iraq, Jordan, Kuwait, Lebanon, Oman, State of Palestine, Qatar, Saudi Arabia, Syrian Arab Republic, United Arab Emirates and Yemen)	• Qatar National Research Fund • Medical Research Centre, Hamad • King Abdulaziz City for Science and Technology, United National Platform
Southeast Asia (Brunei, Burma, Cambodia, Timor-Leste, Indonesia, Laos, Malaysia, Philippines, Singapore, Thailand and Vietnam)	• SEAOHUN—Southeast Asia One Health University Network • SHAPE-SEA's—Strengthening Human Rights and Peace Research and Education in ASEAN/Southeast Asia • Association of Southeast Asian Nations (ASEAN) • E-ASIA Joint Research Program • Bicol Consortium for Health Research and Development, Philippines
Southern Asia (Bangladesh, Bhutan, India, Pakistan, Nepal and Sri Lanka)	• The Bangladesh Medical Research Council • Pakistan Health Research Institute • Nepal Health Research Council • Sri Lanka Medical Association • Indian Council of Medical Research, New Delhi • Department of Science and Technology, New Delhi • Department of Biotechnology

The research grant's central concept should be based on the call's requirements. It should be precise and clear. In most Asian countries, the request for proposals is focused on a pressing health issue that affects the region. As a result, it is critical to

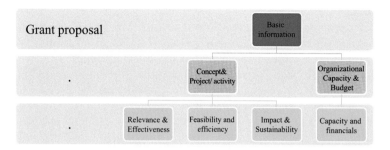

Fig. 21.1 The structure of a regional grant

address the issues raised. The execution method, as well as the expected outcomes and whether they will be meaningful to the general public should all be clearly stated in the proposal. Another aspect to consider is the monitoring and evaluation of the research that will be carried out. The goals should not be too ambitious, keeping in mind the resources at hand. Since funds are limited, the budget must be allocated accordingly. The research should not be a dead-end because the proposal can serve as a framework and foundation for future research (Fig. 21.1). Rejection should not discourage researchers as it allows them to seek out new opportunities, improve their applications and browse the system more effectively [14, 15].

Collaboration is critical and should not be overlooked. Multicentric studies incorporating multiple centers from the same or different regions boost the likelihood of acceptance, while also improving the research outcome. It increases the output and impact of the research conducted. Connecting with others in the same field can help you learn new skills, obtain fresh perspectives and gain insights into new research approaches [16–18].

21.7   Conclusion

Controlling the spread of infectious diseases such as HIV, malaria and zoonotic diseases that cross national borders remains a challenge for Asian countries. Although considerable progress has been made in a few cases and ground-breaking research is also being conducted in a few Asian countries for example, China, which has been declared malaria-free, there is still a long way to go. Research is a never-ending process that improves over time. Promoting regional grants Institute-funded research is one step in that direction, as it opens new doors for researchers as well as the funding agency in the form of new partners and investors.

Case Scenario

1) A call for proposals has been issued by the Health Ministry of your region. The core concept of the proposal is drug resistance in malaria. Therefore, you are required to write a proposal that addresses the following points:

   a) Current state of malarial parasite in your region (Prevalence and Epidemiology) and the status of drug resistance, for example, species against which the drug resistance has been reported

   b) On what particular aspect you would you like your research to be focused

   New methods to identify the drug resistance (molecular methods/sequencing)—the gene involved, identification of SNPs, etc.

   Drug resistance in different *Plasmodium* species (*Plasmodium vivax*, *Plasmodium ovale*, etc.)

   In silico, in vitro and in vivo evaluation of repurposed drugs (drug development)

   Has any similar kind of drug resistance been reported in some other region? If yes, then you can opt for a multi-centric study design.

2) Recently, outbreaks due to a certain bacterium has been reported in your region, write down a proposal for the development of a point-of-care diagnostic test for its identification keeping in mind the resources at hand.

References

1. Meo SA, Sattar K, Ullah CH, Alnassar S, Hajjar W, Usmani AM. Progress and prospects of medical education research in Asian Countries. Pak J Med Sci. 2019;35(6):1475–81.
2. nationsonline.org klaus kästle. List of Asian Countries—Nations Online Project [Internet]. https://www.nationsonline.org/oneworld/asia.htm. Accessed 18 May 2022.
3. Sadana R, D'Souza C, Hyder AA, Chowdhury AMR. Importance of health research in South Asia. BMJ. 2004;328(7443):826–30.
4. Bennett R. Federal grant funding: types and best opportunities. https://www.amplifund.com/blog/federal-grant-funding. Accessed 21 May 2022.
5. NIDCD. Understanding Types of Grants and Funding [Internet]. https://www.nidcd.nih.gov/funding/types. Accessed 21 May 2022.
6. World RePORT: International Biomedical Research Organization Support [Internet]. https://worldreport.nih.gov/wrapp/#/search?searchId=628498a2fe43c863cea96d70.   Accessed 18 May 2022.
7. Research Website [Internet]. https://www.cmch-vellore.edu/sites/research/International%20Funding%20Agencies.html. Accessed 18 May 2022.
8. Small Grants | Southeast Asia One Health University Network | Thailand [Internet]. SEAOHUN.org. https://www.seaohun.org/small-grants. Accessed 21 May 2022.
9. Homepage—Portal RFBR [Internet]. https://www.rfbr.ru/rffi/eng. Accessed 21 May 2022.
10. National Natural Science Foundation of China [Internet]. https://www.nsfc.gov.cn/english/site_1/index.html. Accessed 21 May 2022.
11. Global Health | Asia Regional | U.S. Agency for International Development [Internet]. 2019. https://www.usaid.gov/asia-regional/global-health. Accessed 20 May 2022.
12. About AMED [Internet]. Japan Agency for Medical Research and Development. https://www.amed.go.jp/en/aboutus/index.html. Accessed 21 May 2022.
13. Qatar National Research Fund > Home [Internet]. https://www.qnrf.org/en-us/. Accessed 21 May 2022.

14. Official Website of Bangladesh Medical Research Council (BMRC) [Internet]. https://www.bmrcbd.org/. Accessed 21 May 2022.
15. Sohn E. Secrets to writing a winning grant. Nature. 2019;577(7788):133–5. https://doi.org/10.1038/d41586-019-03914-5.
16. Top 20 Tips for Successful Grant Application [Internet]. Enago Academy 2018. https://www.enago.com/academy/top-20-tips-for-a-successful-grant-application/. Accessed 20 May 2022.
17. 5 ways that collaboration can further your research and your career | For Researchers | Springer Nature [Internet]. https://www.springernature.com/gp/researchers/the-source/blog/blogposts-life-in-research/benefits-of-research-collaboration/17360752. Accessed 20 May 2022.
18. Global Health | Asia Regional | U.S. Agency for International Development [Internet]. https://www.usaid.gov/asia-regional/global-health. Accessed 20 May 2022.

Printed in the United States
by Baker & Taylor Publisher Services